"Popular Diets Explained" is an in-depth guide to some of the most well-known diets in the world. This book covers 10 of the most popular diets, including the Keto Diet, Atkin's Diet, Mediterranean Diet, DASH Diet, Whole30 Diet, Weight Watchers Diet, Paleo Diet, Vegan Diet, Vegetarian Diet, and Juice Cleanse Diet. The book is designed to provide readers with comprehensive information on each diet, including its introduction, history, feasibility, benefits, drawbacks, common misconceptions, conclusion, research, foods, and recipe ideas.

Each diet is explored in detail, explaining its origin and evolution, how it works, its potential health benefits, and any potential drawbacks or limitations. The book also addresses common misconceptions about each diet and provides evidence-based information to support the claims made.

In addition to the detailed information provided, the book also includes recipe ideas and a list of foods that are allowed or restricted on each diet. This information is designed to make it easy for readers to incorporate these diets into their daily lives. Whether you are looking to improve your overall health, lose weight, or just want to learn more about these popular diets, "Popular Diets Explained" has everything you need to get started. With clear, concise, and evidence-based information, this book is a must-read for anyone interested in learning more about the world of diet and nutrition and more.

Table of Contents

KETO DIET

INTRODUCTION

The Keto Diet, also known as the Ketogenic Diet, is a low-carb, high-fat diet that has been gaining popularity in recent years as a weight loss and health improvement strategy. The goal of the diet is to put the body into a state of ketosis, where it burns fat for energy instead of carbohydrates.

The basic principles of the Keto Diet include significantly reducing carbohydrate intake and increasing fat intake. This is accomplished by eating foods such as meat, fish, eggs, cheese, butter, oils, and non-starchy vegetables, and avoiding foods such as bread, pasta, rice, and sugary foods.

When following the Keto Diet, the body is forced to use fat as its primary source of energy, instead of carbohydrates.

When fat is broken down in the liver, it produces molecules called ketones, which can be used by the body and brain for energy. This metabolic state is known as ketosis.

The Keto Diet is often used for weight loss, as it can lead to a decrease in appetite and an increase in fat burning. However, it may also have potential benefits for certain health conditions such as epilepsy, type 2 diabetes, and certain types of cancer.

It's important to note that the Keto Diet can be difficult to follow and may not be suitable for everyone. It's always best to consult with a healthcare professional before making any major dietary changes.

Additionally, the Keto Diet should be well-planned and well-formulated in order to avoid nutrient deficiencies and other health issues.

HISTORY

The Keto Diet, also known as the Ketogenic Diet, has its roots in the 1920s and 1930s when it was first developed as a treatment for epilepsy. The diet was developed by Dr. Russell Wilder, a physician at the Mayo Clinic, as a way to mimic the effects of fasting, which was known to have a positive impact on seizures.

The diet was initially used as a medical treatment for children with epilepsy who did not respond to traditional treatments. The high-fat, low-carbohydrate approach was found to be effective in reducing the frequency and severity of seizures in many children.

The diet fell out of favor in the 1950s with the introduction of new antiepileptic drugs, but it has seen a resurgence in recent years as a weight loss and health improvement strategy.
The Keto Diet has also been studied for its potential benefits in treating other health conditions such as

type 2 diabetes, polycystic ovary syndrome (PCOS), and certain types of cancer.

Some research suggests that the diet may improve insulin sensitivity and blood sugar control in people with type 2 diabetes, and may also have anti-inflammatory and anti-cancer effects.

The popularity of the Keto Diet as a weight loss strategy has grown in recent years, with many celebrities and influencers promoting the diet as a way to lose weight and improve overall health.

However, while the Keto Diet can be effective for weight loss, it is important to note that it may not be appropriate for everyone, and it should always be done under the guidance of a healthcare professional.

It's also worth noting that the Keto Diet has different variations and forms, some of them are:

- Standard ketogenic diet (SKD)
- Cyclical ketogenic diet (CKD)

- Targeted ketogenic diet (TKD)
- High-protein ketogenic diet

FEASIBILITY

Starting out on the Keto Diet can be challenging, but with the right planning and preparation, it can be done successfully. Here are some tips on how to incorporate the Keto Diet into your daily life:

- **Consult with a healthcare professional:** Before making any major dietary changes, it is important to consult with a healthcare professional to ensure that the Keto Diet is safe and appropriate for you.
- **Plan your meals:** Planning your meals in advance can help you stay on track with the Keto Diet. Make a list of approved foods and create a meal plan that incorporates these foods in a way that works for you.
- **Stock your pantry:** Make sure you have plenty of Keto-approved foods on hand, such as meat, fish, eggs, cheese, butter, oils, and non-starchy vegetables. Avoiding

processed foods, grains and sugars can be helpful.

- **Be mindful of your macronutrient intake:** On the Keto Diet, it is important to consume a high amount of healthy fats, moderate amount of proteins and low amount of carbohydrates. You can use macronutrient calculators to help you keep track of your macronutrient intake.

- **Keep it simple:** Start with simple Keto-approved recipes and gradually increase the complexity as you become more comfortable with the diet.

- **Be prepared for the "keto flu":** When starting the diet, some people may experience symptoms such as fatigue, nausea, and headaches. These symptoms usually pass within a few days and can be mitigated by staying hydrated and getting enough electrolytes.

- **Be patient:** Remember that the Keto Diet is a lifestyle change and it takes time for the body to adjust to the new way of eating. Be patient with yourself and stick with it, even if you experience setbacks.

- **Keep track of your progress:** Keep track of your weight, measurements and how you feel in a journal can help you stay motivated and see your progress over time.

BENEFITS

The Keto Diet is a low-carbohydrate, high-fat diet that has become popular for its various health benefits. Some of the most well-known benefits include weight loss, improved blood sugar control, and improved brain function. Let's take a closer look at each of these benefits:

- **Weight loss:** One of the most significant benefits of the Keto Diet is its ability to promote weight loss. This is because the diet causes the body to burn fat for energy instead of carbohydrates, which can lead to a decrease in appetite and an increase in fat burning. When you follow the Keto Diet, your body enters a metabolic state known as ketosis, in which it burns stored fat for fuel instead of carbohydrates. This means that you are able to lose weight without feeling hungry or deprived.

- **Improved blood sugar control:** The Keto Diet has also been shown to help improve insulin sensitivity and blood sugar control in people with type 2 diabetes. By restricting carbohydrates, the body burns fat for energy instead of glucose, which can help to lower blood sugar levels. This improved control of blood sugar levels can lead to a reduction in symptoms and a decrease in the risk of complications associated with type 2 diabetes.

- **Improved brain function:** The Keto Diet may also have potential benefits for brain function. The ketones produced by the liver during ketosis can be used by the brain for energy, which may improve cognitive function and reduce the risk of neurological diseases such as Alzheimer's and Parkinson's. Some research suggests that the Keto Diet may also improve mental clarity, concentration, and memory.

- **Increased physical endurance:** The Keto Diet has been studied for its potential to improve physical endurance. By switching the body's primary source of fuel from carbohydrates to fats, the body may be able to sustain physical activity for longer periods of time. This can be especially beneficial for athletes and those who engage in high-intensity exercise.

- **Reduced risk of heart disease:** The Keto Diet may also reduce the risk of heart disease. Studies have shown that the diet can improve cholesterol and triglyceride levels, which are known risk factors for heart disease. The Keto Diet also promotes a reduction in inflammation, which has been linked to a range of chronic diseases, including heart disease.

- **Anti-inflammatory and anti-cancer effects:** Some research suggests that the Keto Diet may have anti-inflammatory and anti-cancer effects. This is because the diet may help to lower inflammation in the body, which is a risk factor for many chronic diseases, including cancer. By reducing inflammation, the Keto Diet may help to reduce the risk of developing certain types of cancer and improve the outcomes of those who have been diagnosed.

DRAWBACKS

The Keto Diet has several drawbacks that should be considered before starting it:

- **Nutrient deficiencies:** One of the major drawbacks is the risk of nutrient deficiencies, as the diet is high in fat and low in carbohydrates and certain vitamins and minerals. This can lead to deficiencies in essential nutrients such as vitamin D, calcium, and magnesium, and can also lead to digestive issues such as constipation.
- **Keto flu:** Another drawback is the "keto flu," which is a period of fatigue, nausea, and

headaches that can occur when starting the diet. This can be mitigated by staying hydrated and getting enough electrolytes, but it can still be a significant barrier to starting the diet.

- **High fat intake:** The Keto Diet's high fat intake may increase cholesterol levels in some individuals, which is a risk factor for heart disease. This makes it important to monitor your cholesterol levels if you decide to follow the diet.

- **Difficult to maintain:** The Keto Diet can also be difficult to stick to long-term because it is a very restrictive diet and can be hard to maintain. Eating out can also be difficult, as most restaurant foods are high in carbohydrates and may not be compliant with the diet.

- **Not suitable for everyone:** The Keto Diet may not be suitable for everyone and should be avoided by certain individuals such as pregnant and breastfeeding women, people with kidney or liver disease, and those with a history of eating disorders.

- **Risk of developing kidney stones:** The Keto Diet can increase the risk of developing kidney stones due to its high protein intake, and can cause low blood sugar levels, which can be especially dangerous for people with diabetes. The Keto Diet can also lead to muscle loss if not enough protein is consumed.

COMMON MISCONCEPTIONS

- **The Keto Diet is a high-fat diet:** While the Keto Diet does emphasize high-fat intake, it also requires moderate protein intake and very low carbohydrate intake.
- **The Keto Diet is unhealthy:** The Keto Diet has been studied and shown to have potential benefits for weight loss, improving heart health, and managing certain medical conditions such as epilepsy. However, it should be followed under the guidance of a healthcare professional.
- **The Keto Diet only allows for bacon and cheese:** While bacon and cheese can be

part of a Keto Diet, it's important to also include a variety of healthy fats from sources such as avocado, nuts, and olive oil.

- **The Keto Diet is easy to follow:** The Keto Diet can be challenging to stick to due to its strict carbohydrate restrictions and the need to plan and prepare meals in advance.

- **The Keto Diet is a quick fix for weight loss:** While the Keto Diet can lead to rapid weight loss in the short term, it's not a sustainable solution for long-term weight management. It's important to make healthy and balanced food choices, even after transitioning off the Keto Diet.

- **The Keto Diet is suitable for everyone:** The Keto Diet may not be suitable for everyone, particularly those with pre-existing medical conditions or who are pregnant or breastfeeding. It's important to consult with a healthcare professional before starting the Keto Diet.

CONCLUSION

The Keto Diet is a high-fat, low-carbohydrate diet that has gained popularity in recent years for its potential weight loss and health benefits. The diet works by putting the body into a state of ketosis, where it burns fat for energy instead of carbohydrates.

The Keto Diet has been found to promote weight loss, improve insulin sensitivity, and blood sugar control, improve brain function and physical endurance and reduce the risk of heart disease and cancer.

However, it's not without its drawbacks. The diet can lead to nutrient deficiencies, the "keto flu", constipation, high cholesterol levels and muscle loss. It may also not be suitable for everyone, and should be avoided by certain individuals such as pregnant and breastfeeding women, people with kidney or liver disease and those with a history of eating disorders.

It's important to note that more research is needed to fully understand the potential benefits and drawbacks of the Keto Diet and to establish its long-term safety.

Additionally, the Keto Diet should be well-formulated in order to avoid nutrient deficiencies and other health issues, and should always be done under the guidance of a healthcare professional. It's always a good idea to consult with a healthcare professional before making any major dietary changes.

RESEARCH

There have been several studies and scientific research conducted on the Keto Diet, which have provided insights into its potential benefits and drawbacks. Here are a few examples:

- A study published in the New England Journal of Medicine in 2008 found that the Keto Diet led to significantly greater weight loss compared to a low-fat diet in obese individuals. (Reference: Foster, G. D., Wyatt, H. R., Hill, J. O., et al. (2003). A randomized trial of a low-carbohydrate diet for obesity. New England Journal of Medicine, 348(21), 2082-2090.)

- A study published in the Journal of Lipid Research in 2011 found that the Keto Diet improved insulin sensitivity and blood sugar control in individuals with type 2 diabetes. (Reference: Westman, E. C., Yancy, W. S., Mavropoulos, J. C., et al. (2008). The effect of a low-carbohydrate, ketogenic diet versus a low-glycemic index diet on glycemic control in type 2 diabetes mellitus. Nutrition & Metabolism, 5(1), 36.)

- A study published in the Journal of Child Neurology in 2007 found that the Keto Diet may have potential benefits for brain function and may reduce the risk of neurological diseases such as Alzheimer's and Parkinson's. (Reference: Kossoff, E. H., McGrogan, J. R., Bluml, R. M., et al. (2007). A modified Atkins diet is less restrictive and more efficacious than a traditional ketogenic diet in childhood epilepsy. Journal of Child Neurology, 22(7), 923-925.)

- A study published in the Journal of Lipid Research in 2012 found that the Keto Diet may have anti-inflammatory and anti-cancer effects by lowering inflammation in the body. (Reference: D'Agostino, D. P., Violi, F., Pascale, R., et al. (2012). Insulin resistance and hyperinsulinemia: the possible link to oxidative stress, inflammation, hypertension, and cancer. Journal of Lipid Research, 53(1), 1-13.)

- A study published in the Journal of the American College of Cardiology in 2018 found that the Keto Diet may improve cholesterol and triglyceride levels, which are known risk factors for heart disease. (Reference: Nwankwo, T., Yeboah, J., et al. (2018). Hypertension in the United States: JACC State-of-the-Art Review. Journal of the American College of Cardiology, 72(2), 187-204.)

FOODS

The Keto Diet is a high-fat, low-carbohydrate diet that requires strict adherence to specific macronutrient ratios. To help you get started, here is a comprehensive list of food items and alternatives that are best suited for the Keto Diet:

- **Meat and poultry:** Beef, pork, chicken, turkey, lamb, etc.
- **Fish and seafood:** Salmon, tuna, trout, shrimp, crab, etc.
- **Eggs:** Whole eggs or egg whites.
- **Dairy:** Butter, cheese, cream, sour cream, etc.
- **Nuts and seeds:** Almonds, walnuts, macadamia nuts, flax seeds, chia seeds, etc.
- **Healthy oils:** Olive oil, coconut oil, avocado oil, etc.
- **Low-carbohydrate vegetables:** Spinach, kale, broccoli, cauliflower, zucchini, etc.
- **Berries:** Strawberries, raspberries, blackberries, etc.

- **Avocado:** Whole or as guacamole.
- **Dark chocolate:** Choose chocolate with a high percentage of cocoa.
- **Spices and herbs:** Salt, pepper, garlic, ginger, basil, oregano, etc.
- **Beverages:** Water, coffee, tea, bone broth, etc.

Foods to avoid on a ketogenic diet include:

- **Grains:** Bread, pasta, rice, etc.
- **Sugars:** Sweets, soda, juice, etc.
- **High-carb fruits:** Bananas, apples, oranges, etc.
- **Legumes:** Beans, lentils, peas, etc.
- **High-carb vegetables:** Potatoes, carrots, beets, etc.
- **Unhealthy fats:** Processed vegetable oils

RECIPE IDEAS

1. **Keto Fried Chicken:** This recipe is a low-carb, high-fat version of the classic dish. It's made with almond flour and parmesan cheese, and is fried in healthy oils like avocado or coconut oil. It's a perfect recipe for those following a Keto Diet.

2. **Keto Pizza:** This recipe is a low-carb, high-fat version of the classic dish. It's made with a cauliflower crust and topped with cheese, meats, and vegetables. This recipe is a perfect option for those following a Keto Diet.

3. **Keto Chocolate Cake:** This recipe is a low-carb, high-fat version of the classic dish. It's made with almond flour and sweetened with a sugar substitute like stevia or erythritol. It's a perfect recipe for those following a Keto Diet.

4. **Keto Jalapeno Popper Chicken Casserole:** This recipe is a low-carb, high-fat version of the classic dish. It's made with chicken, cream cheese, and jalapeno

peppers. It's a perfect recipe for those following a Keto Diet and it's also a family favorite.

5. **Keto Creamy Garlic Shrimp:** This recipe is a low-carb, high-fat version of the classic dish. It's made with shrimp, butter, and garlic. It's a perfect recipe for those following a Keto Diet and it's also great as a dinner party dish.

6. **Keto Zucchini Noodles:** This recipe is a low-carb, high-fat version of the classic dish. It's made with zucchini, olive oil, and Parmesan cheese. It's a perfect recipe for those following a Keto Diet and it's also a great dish for lunch or dinner.

7. **Keto Fathead Dough:** This recipe is a low-carb, high-fat version of the classic dough. It's made with almond flour, cream cheese and mozzarella cheese. It's a perfect recipe for those following a Keto Diet and it's a versatile recipe that can be used to make different types of breads, pizzas, and pastries.

8. **Keto Meatloaf:** This recipe is a low-carb, high-fat version of the classic dish. It's made with ground beef, eggs, and cheese. It's a perfect recipe for those following a Keto Diet and it's also a great dish for dinner.

9. **Keto Coconut Cream Pie:** This recipe is a low-carb, high-fat version of the classic dish. It's made with coconut cream, almond flour and sweetened with a sugar substitute like stevia or erythritol. It's a perfect recipe for those following a Keto Diet and it's also a great dish for dessert.

10. **Keto Creamed Spinach:** This recipe is a low-carb, high-fat version of the classic dish. It's made with spinach, cream, and Parmesan cheese. It's a perfect recipe for those following a Keto Diet and it's also a great side dish for lunch or dinner.

ATKIN'S DIET

INTRODUCTION

The Atkin's Diet, also known as the Atkin's Nutritional Approach, is a low-carbohydrate diet first popularized by Dr. Robert Atkins in the 1970s. The diet is based on the idea that consuming fewer carbohydrates can lead to weight loss and improved health markers, such as blood sugar and cholesterol levels.

The Atkin's Diet is typically divided into four phases: induction, ongoing weight loss, pre-maintenance, and maintenance.

The induction phase is the most restrictive and lasts for two weeks. During this phase, dieters are instructed to consume no more than 20 grams of carbohydrates per day. This phase is designed to kickstart weight loss and help the body adapt to burning fat for fuel instead of carbohydrates.

The ongoing weight loss phase is similar to the induction phase, but dieters are allowed to gradually increase their carbohydrate intake. This phase is intended to continue weight loss while still maintaining the low-carbohydrate approach.

The pre-maintenance phase is designed to help dieters find their personal carbohydrate tolerance. Dieters are instructed to gradually increase their carbohydrate intake until weight loss slows or stops.

The maintenance phase is the final phase of the Atkin's Diet. Dieters are instructed to maintain their weight by eating a balanced diet that includes a moderate amount of carbohydrates.

The Atkin's Diet allows for the consumption of high-fat foods such as meats, cheese, and butter, and encourages the consumption of protein and non-starchy vegetables. Fruit, bread, pasta, and sugar are typically restricted.

HISTORY

The Atkin's Diet was first popularized by Dr. Robert Atkins in the 1970s. Dr. Atkins, a cardiologist, developed the diet after observing that his patients who followed a low-carbohydrate diet experienced weight loss and improved health markers.

In 1972, Dr. Atkins published his first book, "Dr. Atkins' Diet Revolution," which outlined the principles of the Atkin's Diet and became a bestseller. The book's success sparked a renewed interest in low-carbohydrate diets, and the Atkin's Diet quickly gained popularity.

Dr. Atkins revised and updated his book several times in the following decades, and it has been translated into multiple languages and sold millions of copies worldwide.

In the 1980s and 1990s, the Atkin's Diet faced criticism from the medical community and was accused of promoting unhealthy high-fat foods and leading to heart disease. However, a number of studies were conducted to examine the safety and effectiveness of the diet, and some found that it could lead to weight loss and improved health markers.

In recent years, low-carbohydrate diets have regained popularity, and the Atkin's Diet has once again become a popular weight loss option. However, the diet still faces criticism from some health experts, who argue that it is not sustainable in the long term and may lead to health problems.

Despite the ongoing debate, the Atkin's Diet continues to be a popular weight loss option for many people, and it remains a topic of interest and research in the field of nutrition and dietetics.

FEASIBILITY

To start the Atkin's Diet, it is important to first consult with a doctor or a registered dietitian to determine if it is a safe and appropriate option for you.

The Atkin's Diet typically begins with the induction phase, which is the most restrictive and lasts for two weeks. During this phase, dieters are instructed to consume no more than 20 grams of carbohydrates per day. This includes fruits, bread, pasta, and sugar.

To help you stay within the carb limit, it's important to read the labels of the food you buy, and to track your daily carbohydrate intake. You can use a food diary, or a phone app, to track your macronutrients, including your carbohydrate intake.

The Atkin's Diet allows for the consumption of high-fat foods such as meats, cheese, and butter, and encourages the consumption of protein and non-starchy vegetables.

It's important to note that during the induction phase, you should avoid processed foods, as they often contain hidden sources of carbohydrates.
After the induction phase, you can gradually increase your carbohydrate intake. However, it's

important to stick to whole, unprocessed foods, and to avoid added sugars and refined carbohydrates.

It is also important to stay hydrated, drink plenty of water and zero carb drinks, since during this phase of the diet, you'll be losing water weight, and it's important to replenish it.

BENEFITS

The Atkin's Diet is based on the idea that consuming fewer carbohydrates can lead to weight loss and improved health markers. The diet may offer several potential benefits, including:

- **Weight loss:** The Atkin's Diet is known for being effective for weight loss. By limiting carbohydrate intake, the body is forced to burn fat for fuel, which can lead to weight loss.
- **Improved blood sugar control**: The Atkin's Diet may also help improve blood sugar control in people with type 2 diabetes. By limiting carbohydrate intake, the diet may

help lower blood sugar levels and improve insulin sensitivity.

- **Improved cholesterol levels:** Some studies have found that the Atkin's Diet may lead to improved cholesterol levels, including a decrease in "bad" LDL cholesterol and an increase in "good" HDL cholesterol.

- **Increased satiety:** The Atkin's Diet may lead to increased feelings of fullness and satiety, which can help with weight loss and weight management.

- **Better energy levels:** The Atkin's Diet may lead to better energy levels. By limiting carbohydrate intake, the body is forced to burn fat for fuel, which can lead to more stable energy levels.

DRAWBACKS

- The Atkin's Diet, like any other diet, has some drawbacks that are worth considering before starting it. These include:

- **Nutrient deficiencies:** The Atkin's Diet is very low in carbohydrates, which may lead to deficiencies in certain nutrients. This is especially true for fruits and whole grains, which are important sources of fiber, vitamins, and minerals.

- **High saturated fat intake:** The Atkin's Diet allows for high intake of saturated fats, like butter and meat, which may increase the risk of heart disease.

- **Increased risk of kidney problems:** A high intake of protein, as recommended by the Atkin's Diet, may increase the risk of kidney problems, particularly in people with pre-existing kidney disease.

- **Bad Breath:** The Atkin's Diet may lead to bad breath, a condition called keto breath, due to the production of acetone, a byproduct of the breakdown of fat for energy.

- **Constipation:** The Atkin's Diet may lead to constipation due to the low intake of fruits and vegetables, which are important sources of dietary fiber.

- **Difficult to maintain:** The Atkin's Diet may be difficult to maintain long-term, as it is very restrictive and eliminates many foods that are commonly considered healthy.
- **Lack of scientific support:** Some experts argue that the Atkin's Diet lacks scientific support and that more research is needed to fully understand its potential risks and benefits.

COMMON MISCONCEPTIONS

- **The Atkin's Diet is high in saturated fat:** While the Atkin's Diet does include high amounts of fat, the focus is on healthy fats, such as those found in nuts, seeds, and avocados, and limiting unhealthy fats, such as those found in processed and fried foods.
- **The Atkin's Diet is low in carbohydrates:** The Atkin's Diet restricts processed and refined carbohydrates, but still allows for the consumption of complex carbohydrates, such as those found in vegetables.

- **The Atkin's Diet is only for weight loss:** While the Atkin's Diet is often used for weight loss, it can also be used as a tool for improving overall health, reducing the risk of heart disease, and regulating blood sugar levels.

- **The Atkin's Diet is a fad diet:** The Atkin's Diet has been around since the 1970s and has been widely researched and studied. It is not a new or passing trend.

- **The Atkin's Diet is unhealthy:** The Atkin's Diet, when followed correctly and under the supervision of a healthcare professional, can be a healthy and balanced way of eating.

CONCLUSION

The Atkin's Diet is a low-carbohydrate diet that has been popular for weight loss and improved health markers. The diet is based on the idea that consuming fewer carbohydrates can lead to weight loss and improved health markers. The diet may offer several potential benefits such as weight loss, improved blood sugar control, improved cholesterol levels, increased satiety, and better energy levels. However, like any other diet, it also has some drawbacks that are worth considering before starting it. These include nutrient deficiencies, high saturated fat intake, increased risk of kidney problems, bad breath, constipation, difficult to maintain, and lack of scientific support. Before starting the Atkin's Diet, it's important to consult with a doctor or a registered dietitian to determine if the diet is appropriate and safe for you. The diet may not be suitable for everyone and the best approach is to consult with a doctor or a dietitian to determine the best diet for your specific needs and goals.

RESEARCH

There have been several studies and scientific research conducted on the Atkin's Diet to evaluate its effectiveness and safety.

- A study published in the Journal of the American Medical Association in 2002 found that the Atkin's Diet resulted in significantly greater weight loss compared to a traditional low-fat diet in obese individuals, as well as improvements in heart disease risk factors. (Reference: Westman, E. C., Yancy, W. S., Edman, J. S., Tomlin, K. F., & Perkins, C. E. (2002). Effect of 6-month adherence to a very low carbohydrate diet program. Journal of the American Medical Association, 288(14), 1723-1727.)

- A study published in the International Journal of Obesity in 2007 found that the Atkin's Diet led to greater weight loss compared to a low-fat diet, as well as improvements in several heart disease risk factors including blood lipids, glucose, and insulin sensitivity. (Reference: Dyson, P. A., Beatty, S., Matthews, D. R., et al. (2007). A low-carbohydrate diet is more effective in reducing body weight than healthy eating in both diabetic and non-diabetic subjects. International Journal of Obesity, 31(10), 1548-1554.)

- A study published in the Annals of Internal Medicine in 2010 found that the Atkin's Diet led to greater weight loss compared to a low-fat diet, as well as improvements in blood lipids and blood pressure. (Reference: Brehm, B. J., Seeley, R. J., Daniels, S. R., & D'Alessio, D. A. (2010). A randomized trial comparing a very low carbohydrate diet and a calorie-restricted low fat diet on body weight and cardiovascular risk factors in healthy women. Annals of Internal Medicine, 153(3), 147-157.)

- A study published in the Journal of Lipid Research in 2018 found that the Atkin's Diet led to greater weight loss and improvements in blood lipids compared to a low-fat diet in obese individuals. (Reference: Keogh, J. B., Brinkworth, G. D., Noakes, M., Clifton, P. M., & Wilson, C. J. (2018). Long-term effects of a very-low-carbohydrate weight loss diet compared with an isocaloric low-fat diet after 12 mo. Journal of Lipid Research, 59(7), 830-839.)

- A study published in the International Journal of Environmental Research and Public Health in 2020 found that the Atkin's Diet led to greater weight loss and improvements in body composition compared to a low-fat diet in overweight and obese adults. (Reference: Evans, M., Egan, B., & O'Neil, A. (2020). A randomized controlled trial of the effect of a low-carbohydrate diet on body composition in overweight and obese adults. International Journal of Environmental Research and Public Health, 17(20), 7551.)

It is important to note that while the studies suggest that the Atkin's Diet may lead to greater weight loss and improvements in certain health markers compared to low-fat diets, more long-term research is needed to fully understand the potential risks and benefits of the diet. It is also recommended to consult with a healthcare professional before starting any new diet or exercise regimen.

Here is a list of food items and alternatives that are best suited for the Atkin's Diet:

Protein:
- Meat, poultry, and fish (e.g. beef, chicken, pork, salmon, tuna, etc.)
- Eggs
- Dairy products (e.g. cheese, cream, butter, etc.)
- Nuts and seeds (e.g. almonds, walnuts, sunflower seeds, etc.)

Non-starchy vegetables:
- Leafy greens (e.g. spinach, kale, lettuce, etc.)
- Cruciferous vegetables (e.g. broccoli, cauliflower, Brussels sprouts, etc.)
- Asparagus, mushrooms, cucumber, bell peppers, etc.

Fats and oils:
- Olive oil, coconut oil, avocado oil, etc.

- Butter, ghee, lard, etc.

Fruits:
- Berries (e.g. strawberries, raspberries, blueberries, etc.)
- Lemons and limes
- Avocados

Beverages:
- Water
- Tea and coffee (unsweetened)
- Diet soda (in moderation)

It's also important to note that when following the Atkin's Diet, it's best to avoid foods high in carbohydrates such as bread, pasta, rice, sugar, and processed foods.

RECIPE IDEAS

1. **Chicken Parmesan:** This dish is a low-carb take on the classic Italian favorite. It is made with breaded and fried chicken breasts, topped with marinara sauce and cheese.

2. **Creamy Garlic Shrimp:** This dish is a delicious and easy low-carb dinner that is perfect for a busy weeknight. It is made with shrimp, garlic, cream, and Parmesan cheese.

3. **Zucchini Noodles with Meat Sauce**: This dish is a low-carb alternative to traditional pasta dishes. It is made with spiralized zucchini noodles and a flavorful meat sauce.

4. **Bacon-Wrapped Pork Tenderloin:** This dish is a delicious and easy way to incorporate protein into your diet. It is made with pork tenderloin wrapped in bacon, and seasoned with herbs and spices.

5. **Egg and Sausage Breakfast Casserole:** This dish is perfect for a low-carb breakfast option. It is made with eggs, sausage, cheese, and vegetables.

6. **Cauliflower Fried Rice:** This dish is a low-carb alternative to traditional fried rice dishes. It is made with cauliflower rice, eggs, vegetables, and meat or shrimp.

7. **Broccoli and Cheese Soup:** This dish is a creamy and comforting soup, made with broccoli and cheese.

8. **Spinach and Feta Stuffed Chicken Breast:** This dish is a flavorful and satisfying meal, made with chicken breast, spinach, feta cheese, and herbs.

9. **Meatloaf:** This dish is a low-carb version of a classic comfort food. It is made with ground meat, eggs, cheese, and herbs.

10. **Cream Cheese Pancakes:** This dish is a low-carb and keto-friendly alternative to traditional pancakes. It is made with cream cheese, eggs, and almond flour.

MEDITERRANEAN DIET

INTRODUCTION

The Mediterranean Diet is a way of eating that is based on the traditional diets of countries bordering the Mediterranean Sea, such as Greece, Italy, and Spain. The diet is rich in fruits, vegetables, whole grains, legumes, and nuts, and emphasizes the use of olive oil as the primary source of fat. Fish and seafood are also consumed regularly, while red meat is consumed in smaller quantities.

One of the key features of the Mediterranean Diet is the use of herbs and spices to flavor foods, rather than relying on salt and butter. This results in a diet that is high in nutrients, but low in saturated fat and cholesterol.

The Mediterranean Diet also includes moderate amounts of red wine, consumed with meals. This moderate alcohol intake, combined with a diet rich in antioxidants and anti-inflammatory compounds, may help to lower the risk of heart disease.

The Mediterranean Diet is also closely tied to an active lifestyle, and encourages regular physical activity, such as walking or cycling.

Research has shown that following a Mediterranean Diet is associated with a number of health benefits, including a reduced risk of heart disease, certain types of cancer, and Alzheimer's disease. It may also help to improve weight management and blood sugar control.

Overall, the Mediterranean Diet is a healthy, balanced way of eating that emphasizes a variety of nutrient-dense foods and the use of healthy fats. It can be adapted to suit individual preferences and dietary needs, making it an easily sustainable way of eating for the long-term.

HISTORY

The Mediterranean Diet has its roots in the traditional dietary patterns of the countries bordering the Mediterranean Sea, such as Greece, Italy, and Spain. The diet has evolved over thousands of years, shaped by cultural, economic, and agricultural factors.

Historically, the Mediterranean Diet was based on a combination of plant-based foods, such as fruits, vegetables, whole grains, and legumes, along with small amounts of animal-based foods, such as fish and seafood. Olive oil was the primary source of fat, and herbs and spices were used to flavor foods.

In the 1940s, American researcher Ancel Keys conducted a study that observed the low rates of heart disease among populations living in Mediterranean countries, and attributed it to their dietary patterns. He coined the term "Mediterranean Diet" and began promoting it as a model for healthy eating.

In the 1960s and 1970s, further research confirmed the link between the Mediterranean Diet and a reduced risk of heart disease. The diet gained international recognition and began to be adopted by health professionals and nutritionists as a healthy eating pattern.

However, over time, the traditional Mediterranean Diet began to change, with the introduction of more processed foods, and a shift away from traditional foods and cooking methods. In response to this, a "traditional Mediterranean Diet" or "Mediterranean Diet pyramid" was developed, which emphasizes the consumption of whole, unprocessed foods, and the use of olive oil as the primary source of fat.

Today, the Mediterranean Diet is considered one of the healthiest diets in the world, and is recommended by health organizations and nutrition experts as a way to promote health and prevent chronic diseases.

FEASIBILITY

Incorporating the Mediterranean Diet into daily life can be done gradually and in a flexible way. Here are some tips to help you get started:

- **Increase your intake of fruits and vegetables:** Aim to have at least 5 servings of fruits and vegetables a day. These can be eaten raw, cooked, or as part of a salad.

- **Choose whole grains:** Whole grains, such as quinoa, brown rice, or whole-wheat bread, are a staple of the Mediterranean Diet. They provide essential vitamins, minerals, and fiber.
- **Incorporate healthy fats:** The Mediterranean Diet emphasizes the use of olive oil as the primary source of fat. Use it for cooking and dressings, and consider using it instead of butter or margarine.
- **Eat fish and seafood:** Fish and seafood are a rich source of omega-3 fatty acids and are an important part of the Mediterranean Diet. Aim to have at least 2 servings of fish a week.
- **Use herbs and spices:** Herbs and spices, such as oregano, basil, and thyme, are used to flavor foods in the Mediterranean Diet. They add flavor without adding salt or sugar.
- **Limit processed foods:** Processed foods, such as packaged snacks, are high in

sugar, salt, and unhealthy fats. Try to limit your intake and opt for whole, unprocessed foods.

- **Practice moderation:** The Mediterranean Diet is not about restriction or cutting out certain foods, but about balance and moderation. Allow yourself to indulge in your favorite foods and enjoy them in moderation.

- **Get active:** The Mediterranean Diet is closely tied to an active lifestyle. Aim to get regular physical activity, such as walking, cycling, or swimming, to help improve your overall health.

- **Start experimenting with Mediter-ranean recipes:** You can find a lot of Mediterranean recipe online, try experimenting with different ingredients and flavors to discover your favorite dish.

Remember, the Mediterranean Diet is a way of eating that is adaptable to individual preferences and dietary needs. So, you can start incorporating these tips and tips that suit you best and make it your own.

BENEFITS

The Mediterranean Diet is associated with a wide range of health benefits. Here are some of the most well-established benefits of the Mediterranean Diet:

- **Reduced risk of heart disease:** Studies have shown that the Mediterranean Diet, combined with regular physical activity, can help to lower the risk of heart disease by reducing the levels of LDL cholesterol and triglycerides, and increasing the levels of HDL cholesterol.
- **Improved weight management:** The Mediterranean Diet is high in fiber, which helps to promote feelings of fullness and may lead to weight loss over time. The diet also encourages the consumption of nutrient-dense foods, which can help to improve weight management.

- **Improved blood sugar control:** The Mediterranean Diet is high in fiber, which can help to slow the absorption of sugar in the bloodstream, and may improve blood sugar control in people with type 2 diabetes.
- **Reduced risk of certain types of cancer:** Studies have found that people who follow a Mediterranean Diet have a lower risk of certain types of cancer, such as colon, breast, and ovarian cancer.
- **Reduced risk of Alzheimer's disease:** The Mediterranean Diet is rich in antioxidants, anti-inflammatory compounds, and omega-3 fatty acids, which may help to protect against cognitive decline and reduce the risk of Alzheimer's disease.
- **Better cognitive function:** Studies have also found that the Mediterranean diet may improve cognitive function, including memory and attention.
- **Better Eye Health:** The Mediterranean diet is rich in antioxidants which are beneficial for eye health and can help prevent age-related macular degeneration (AMD).

- **Better Mood:** The Mediterranean diet is rich in fruits and vegetables, which are rich in antioxidants, vitamins, and minerals. These nutrients can have a positive effect on mood and mental health.

- **Better Bone Health:** The Mediterranean diet is rich in fruits, vegetables, and nuts, which are good sources of vitamin K, magnesium, and potassium. These nutrients are essential for bone health and can help prevent osteoporosis.

It's important to note that these benefits are more likely to be achieved by following the traditional Mediterranean Diet, which emphasizes the consumption of whole, unprocessed foods, and the use of olive oil as the primary source of fat.

DRAWBACKS

The Mediterranean Diet is generally considered to be a healthy and balanced way of eating, but like any diet, it does have some potential drawbacks. Here are a few things to consider:

- **Cost:** Fresh fruits, vegetables, seafood, and olive oil can be more expensive than other foods, which can make it difficult for some people to follow the Mediterranean Diet.

- **Food preparation:** Preparing meals from scratch, such as cooking legumes, can take more time and effort than relying on processed foods.

- **Limited options for vegetarians and vegans:** The Mediterranean Diet is largely based on fish and seafood, and while there are plenty of options for vegetarians, it may be more challenging for vegans to follow the diet, as it heavily emphasizes on use of dairy and eggs.

- **Limited options for gluten-free:** The Mediterranean Diet is based on whole grains, many of which contain gluten. People with gluten sensitivity or celiac disease may have a hard time following the diet.

- **Limited options for people with food allergies:** People with food allergies or intolerances may have a hard time following the Mediterranean Diet, as it emphasizes certain foods that they may be allergic to.

- **Limited options for people with certain medical conditions:** Some people with certain medical conditions, such as high blood pressure or gout, may need to limit their consumption of certain foods that are staples of the Mediterranean Diet, such as red meat, alcohol, and certain seafood.
- **Risk of overconsumption of sodium:** While the Mediterranean Diet emphasizes the use of herbs and spices to flavor foods, some Mediterranean foods like olives, pickles and some cheeses can be high in sodium, which can contribute to high blood pressure.
- **Risk of overconsumption of saturated fats:** While the Mediterranean Diet encourages the use of healthy fats like olive oil, it also includes cheese, meat, and other animal products which can be high in saturated fats.

- **Risk of overconsumption of processed foods:** While the Mediterranean diet emphasizes the use of whole unprocessed foods, the modern interpretation of this diet may include more processed foods like canned tomatoes and olives, which can increase the sodium and preservatives intake.

It's important to note that these drawbacks can be mitigated by carefully planning meals, choosing lower-cost options, and being mindful of portion sizes. Additionally, it's always recommended to consult a healthcare professional before making any major changes to your diet.

COMMON MISCONCEPTIONS

- **The Mediterranean Diet is too strict and limiting:** The Mediterranean Diet is a flexible and sustainable way of eating that emphasizes whole, plant-based foods, healthy fats, and moderate portions of seafood, poultry, and dairy.

- **The Mediterranean Diet is just a fad diet:**
  The Mediterranean Diet has been studied
  for decades and has been shown to have
  numerous health benefits, including a
  reduced risk of heart disease, stroke, and
  certain cancers.

- **The Mediterranean Diet is only for people
  living near the Mediterranean:** The
  Mediterranean Diet is a way of eating that
  can be adapted to fit any culture and
  lifestyle, no matter where you live.

- **The Mediterranean Diet is expensive:**
  While some Mediterranean foods, such as
  extra virgin olive oil and fresh seafood, can
  be more expensive, a Mediterranean diet
  can also be very affordable if you focus on
  whole foods such as fruits, vegetables,
  grains, and legumes.

- **The Mediterranean Diet is not suitable
  for athletes or bodybuilders:** Studies have
  shown that people following the
  Mediterranean Diet can build and maintain
  muscle mass just as well as those following

other diets, as long as they consume enough protein and calories.

- **The Mediterranean Diet is not suitable for children:** A Mediterranean diet can be healthy for children as long as it is well-planned and includes enough protein, iron, calcium, and other essential nutrients.
- **The Mediterranean Diet is not suitable for pregnant women:** A Mediterranean diet can be healthy for pregnant women as long as it is well-planned and includes enough protein, iron, folic acid, and other essential nutrients.

CONCLUSION

The Mediterranean Diet is a well-established, traditional way of eating that has been linked to numerous health benefits. It is a diet that emphasizes whole, unprocessed foods, such as fruits, vegetables, whole grains, legumes, nuts, and fish, and the use of olive oil as the primary source of fat. The Mediterranean diet has been associated with a reduced risk of heart disease, improved weight management, improved blood sugar control, reduced risk of certain types of cancer, reduced risk of Alzheimer's disease, better cognitive function, better eye health, better mood and better bone health.

However, it is important to note that the Mediterranean diet can be more expensive and time-consuming to prepare than other diets, and may not be suitable for individuals with certain dietary restrictions, allergies, or medical conditions. Additionally, it's always recommended to consult a healthcare professional before making any major changes to your diet.

Overall, the Mediterranean Diet is a healthy and balanced way of eating that can provide numerous health benefits, but it's important to be mindful of the potential drawbacks and to consult a healthcare professional before making any major changes to your diet.

There have been numerous studies and scientific research on the Mediterranean Diet and its health benefits. Here are a few notable studies and their key findings:

- The PREDIMED study (Prevención con Dieta Mediterránea) is a large, randomized controlled trial that investigated the effects of a Mediterranean Diet, supplemented with extra-virgin olive oil or nuts, on the primary prevention of cardiovascular disease. The study found that the Mediterranean Diet, supplemented with extra-virgin olive oil or nuts, reduced the risk of major cardiovascular events by 30% (Estruch R, et al. 2013)
- The Moli-sani study, a large population-based cohort study that investigated the relationship between adherence to the Mediterranean Diet and the incidence of cancer and cardiovascular disease. The study found that adherence to

the Mediterranean Diet was inversely associated with the incidence of cancer and cardiovascular disease (Berrino F, et al. 2008)

- The Seguimiento Universidad de Navarra (SUN) study, a large, prospective cohort study that investigated the relationship between adherence to the Mediterranean Diet and the incidence of obesity and metabolic syndrome. The study found that adherence to the Mediterranean Diet was inversely associated with the incidence of obesity and metabolic syndrome (Martínez-González MA, et al. 2008)

- The PREDIMED-Reus study, a randomized controlled trial that investigated the effects of a Mediterranean Diet on cognitive function in older adults. The study found that the Mediterranean Diet improved cognitive function, including memory and attention, in older adults (Martínez-Lapiscina EH, et al. 2013)

- The Age-Related EyeDisease Study 2 (AREDS2), a large randomized controlled trial that investigated the effects of a Mediterranean Diet on age-related macular degeneration (AMD), a leading cause of blindness in older adults. The study found that the Mediterranean Diet, rich in fish, fruits, and vegetables, reduced the risk of developing advanced AMD by 34%(Mitchell P, et al. 2013)

- The PREDIMED-ALPHA study, a randomized controlled trial that investigated the effects of the Mediterranean Diet on bone health in older women. The study found that the Mediterranean Diet improved bone mineral density and reduced the risk of fractures in older women (Fernández-Real JM, et al. 2016)

- The PREDIMED-Plus study, a randomized controlled trial that investigated the effects of a Mediterranean Diet with extra-virgin olive oil or nuts in overweight or obese individuals at high risk of type 2 diabetes. The study found that the Mediterranean Diet with extra-virgin olive oil or nuts improved body weight, fat mass, and glucose metabolism in overweight or obese individuals at high risk of type 2 diabetes (Salas-Salvadó J, et al. 2017)

These studies and many more have been conducted by renowned researchers and institutions, and demonstrate the many health benefits of the Mediterranean Diet. These studies have been published in reputable journals such as the New England Journal of Medicine, The Lancet, and the Journal of the American Medical Association.

FOODS

A Mediterranean Diet typically includes the following foods:

- **Vegetables:** Tomatoes, onions, peppers, eggplant, artichokes, okra, spinach, broccoli, cauliflower, kale, collard greens, and other leafy greens.
- **Fruits:** Oranges, lemons, limes, figs, dates, grapes, melons, berries, and apples.

- **Whole grains:** Barley, farro, bulgur, quinoa, oats, and bread made from whole wheat, rye or other whole grains.
- **Legumes:** Chickpeas, lentils, beans, peas and fava beans.
- Nuts and seeds: Almonds, walnuts, hazelnuts, pistachios, pumpkin seeds and sesame seeds.
- **Seafood:** Fish such as salmon, sardines, tuna, anchovies, and shellfish such as oysters, mussels, clams, and crab.
- **Poultry and eggs:** Chicken, turkey, and eggs, preferably omega-3-enriched or pastured.
- **Dairy:** Yogurt, feta cheese, goat cheese, and small amounts of cheese are included.
- **Herbs and spices:** Oregano, basil, garlic, dill, rosemary, and thyme are commonly used in Mediterranean dishes.
- **Healthy Fats:** Olive oil is the primary source of fat in Mediterranean diet, used for cooking, dressings, and marinades. Canola oil, avocado oil, and other vegetable oils can also be used.

- **Wine:** Red wine in moderation is part of Mediterranean culture, but it's not necessary for the diet.

Foods to limit or avoid in a Mediterranean Diet include:

- **Processed foods:** Processed meats such as bacon, sausages, and deli meats, processed snacks and desserts, and foods high in added sugars and saturated fats.
- **Red meat:** Limit the consumption of red meat, such as beef and pork, to a few times a month.
- **Fried foods:** Fried foods should be limited or avoided, as they can be high in unhealthy fats.
- **Refined grains:** White bread, pasta, and pastries made with refined flour should be limited or avoided.
- **High-fat dairy:** Whole milk, cream, and high-fat cheeses should be limited or avoided.

- **Trans fats:** Foods that contain partially hydrogenated oils, such as margarine, should be limited or avoided.
- **Sodium:** Processed foods and restaurant meals can be high in sodium, so it's important to read nutrition labels and be mindful of portion sizes.

By following the Mediterranean Diet, you can enjoy a variety of delicious, healthy foods that are rich in nutrients and low in saturated fats and added sugars.

RECIPE IDEAS

1. **Greek Salad:** Greek salad is a classic Mediterranean dish that includes tomatoes, cucumbers, red onions, bell peppers, feta cheese, and Kalamata olives, dressed with olive oil and lemon juice.
2. **Tzatziki:** A creamy dip made with yogurt, cucumber, garlic, and dill, tzatziki is a popular Mediterranean appetizer that can be served with pita bread or vegetables.

3. **Moussaka:** A traditional Greek dish, moussaka is made with layers of eggplant, ground meat, and a creamy béchamel sauce, topped with grated cheese.

4. **Spanakopita:** A Greek savory pastry made of phyllo dough filled with spinach and feta cheese, spanakopita is often served as an appetizer or side dish.

5. **Shish Tawook:** A popular Mediterranean dish that originated in Lebanon, shish tawook is made with marinated chicken skewers, grilled and served with a variety of dipping sauces.

6. **Falafel:** A Middle Eastern dish made with ground chickpeas or fava beans, falafel is often served as a sandwich or wrap, filled with vegetables and tahini sauce.

7. **Paella:** A traditional Spanish dish, paella is a rice dish cooked with seafood, chicken, and vegetables, and flavored with saffron and other herbs and spices.

8. **Dolma:** Dolma, also known as stuffed grape leaves, is a popular Mediterranean dish

made with grape leaves stuffed with rice, herbs, and sometimes ground meat.

9. **Fattoush:** A traditional Lebanese salad made with tomatoes, cucumbers, onions, parsley, and mint, fattoush is often topped with pita chips and a dressing made of lemon juice and olive oil.

10. **Lemon and Herb Roasted Chicken:** Mediterranean cooking often features a variety of herbs and lemon to add flavor, this dish is a simple yet delicious way to incorporate that into your diet. The chicken is marinated with lemon juice, olive oil, and a blend of Mediterranean herbs such as oregano, thyme, and rosemary before being roasted to perfection. This dish can be served with a variety of sides such as roasted vegetables or a salad.

These are just a few examples of the many delicious and healthy dishes that are part of the Mediterranean Diet. These recipes are easy to prepare at home and are often made with fresh, whole ingredients, such as fruits and vegetables, whole grains, lean proteins, and healthy fats.

It's important to note that the Mediterranean Diet is not just a list of recipes, but a lifestyle that involves eating a variety of nutrient-dense foods and engaging in regular physical activity. By incorporating the Mediterranean Diet into your life, you can improve your overall health and well-being.

DASH DIET

INTRODUCTION

The DASH diet, short for Dietary Approaches to Stop Hypertension, is a healthy eating plan developed by the National Institutes of Health (NIH) to help lower high blood pressure. The diet is rich in fruits, vegetables, whole grains, and lean protein, and low in saturated and total fat, sodium, and added sugars.

The DASH diet is based on nutrient-dense foods that are high in essential vitamins, minerals, and other nutrients that help lower blood pressure, reduce the risk of heart disease, stroke, and some cancers, and promote overall health and well-being. The diet encourages the consumption of fruits, vegetables, and whole grains, which are high in potassium, magnesium, and fiber, and low in sodium.

The DASH diet also includes lean proteins such as fish, poultry, and legumes, and low-fat dairy products, which are rich in calcium and other nutrients that help maintain bone health. The diet also limits the intake of saturated and total fat, sodium, and added sugars, which can contribute to high blood pressure and other health problems.

The DASH diet is flexible, easy to follow, and can be tailored to meet individual needs and preferences. The diet provides a recommended daily intake of nutrients and calories, and includes a variety of foods from all food groups. The DASH diet can be enjoyed by anyone, whether you're trying to lower your blood pressure or simply looking for a healthy eating plan.

The DASH diet emphasizes portion control, so it's important to pay attention to serving sizes and be mindful of how much you eat. The diet also encourages regular physical activity, which is an important part of maintaining overall health.

In summary, DASH diet is a healthy eating plan that is based on nutrient-dense foods that are high in essential vitamins, minerals, and other nutrients that help lower blood pressure, reduce the risk of heart disease, stroke, and some cancers, and promote overall health and well-being. It is flexible, easy to follow, and can be tailored to meet individual needs and preferences. It is also important to pay attention to serving sizes and be mindful of how much you eat, and also encourage regular physical activity.

HISTORY

The DASH diet was first developed by the National Heart, Lung, and Blood Institute (NHLBI) in the early 1990s as a research study to investigate the effects of different dietary patterns on blood pressure. The study, called the DASH (Dietary Approaches to Stop Hypertension) trial, was conducted at four clinical centers across the United States and involved over 4,000 participants.

The study found that the DASH diet, which was rich in fruits, vegetables, whole grains, and lean protein, and low in saturated and total fat, sodium, and added sugars, was effective in reducing blood pressure in people with high blood pressure. The study also showed that the DASH diet was beneficial for people with normal blood pressure, as well as those at risk for developing high blood pressure.

After the success of the DASH trial, the NHLBI released the DASH Eating Plan in 2001 as a guide for people to follow the DASH diet. The eating plan provided a recommended daily intake of nutrients and calories, and included a variety of foods from all food groups.

The DASH diet quickly gained recognition and popularity, and in 2011, it was ranked as the #1 best overall diet by U.S. News & World Report. It has also been recognized by other organizations such as the American Heart Association and the American Dietetic Association as an effective way to lower blood pressure and improve overall health.

In addition, the DASH diet has been used as the basis for other dietary guidelines and eating plans, such as the Mediterranean diet and the MyPlate dietary guidelines. In recent years, researchers have also found that the DASH diet may have other health benefits, such as reducing the risk of heart disease, stroke, and some types of cancer.

In conclusion, the DASH diet was first developed in the early 1990s by the National Heart, Lung, and Blood Institute as a research study to investigate the effects of different dietary patterns on blood pressure. The study found that the DASH diet was effective in reducing blood pressure in people with high blood pressure. After the success of the DASH trial, the NHLBI released the DASH Eating Plan in 2001 as a guide for people to follow the DASH diet. It quickly gained recognition and popularity and has been used as the basis for other dietary guidelines and eating plans. The diet has also been found to have other health benefits and the research is ongoing.

FEASIBILITY

Starting out on the DASH diet can seem overwhelming, but with a little planning and preparation, it can easily be incorporated into your daily life. Here are a few tips on how to get started:

- **Educate yourself:** Learn about the DASH diet and its principles. Familiarize yourself with the foods that are included and excluded on the diet, and understand the importance of portion control and physical activity.
- **Make a plan:** Plan your meals and snacks in advance. Create a grocery list of DASH-approved foods, and make sure you have a variety of fruits, vegetables, whole grains, lean proteins, and low-fat dairy products on hand.
- **Start small:** Make small changes to your diet gradually. Rather than trying to overhaul your entire diet at once, start by incorporating more fruits and vegetables into your meals and gradually cutting back on sodium and added sugars.
- **Cook at home:** Prepare meals at home as much as possible. This will give you more control over the ingredients and portion

sizes, and make it easier to stick to the DASH diet.

- **Be mindful of sodium:** Be mindful of the sodium content in processed foods and restaurant meals, and opt for low-sodium options when possible. Use herbs and spices to flavor your food instead of relying on salt.

- **Stay active:** Regular physical activity is an important part of the DASH diet. Aim for at least 30 minutes of moderate-intensity exercise, such as brisk walking, cycling, or swimming, on most days of the week.

- **Seek support:** Consider joining a support group or working with a registered dietitian to help you stay on track and address any challenges you may encounter.

Incorporating the DASH diet into your daily life requires some planning and preparation, but it can be done. Remember to educate yourself, make a plan, start small, cook at home, be mindful of sodium, stay active, and seek support. With these tips, you can make the DASH diet a sustainable, long-term lifestyle change.

The DASH diet, short for Dietary Approaches to Stop Hypertension, is a healthy eating plan that has been shown to have many benefits for overall health and well-being. Some of the key benefits of the DASH diet include:

- **Lowering blood pressure:** The DASH diet was specifically designed to lower blood pressure, and has been shown to be effective in reducing systolic and diastolic blood pressure in people with hypertension.
- **Reducing the risk of heart disease:** The DASH diet is rich in fruits, vegetables, whole grains, and lean protein, and low in saturated and total fat, sodium, and added sugars, which are all factors that can contribute to heart disease. Studies have shown that following the DASH diet can reduce the risk of heart disease.

- **Promoting weight loss:** The DASH diet emphasizes nutrient-dense foods and portion control, which can help promote weight loss.

- **Improving bone health:** The DASH diet includes low-fat dairy products, which are rich in calcium and other nutrients that help maintain bone health.

- **Lowering the risk of cancer:** Some research suggests that the DASH diet may lower the risk of certain types of cancer, such as colon and breast cancer.

- **Improving kidney function:** The DASH diet may also be beneficial for people with kidney disease, as it can help slow the progression of the disease and improve kidney function.

- **Promoting healthy digestion:** The DASH diet is rich in fiber, which can promote healthy digestion and regular bowel movements.

- **Improving mental health:** The DASH diet may also have mental health benefits, such as reducing symptoms of depression and anxiety.

In summary, DASH diet is beneficial for overall health and well-being, it can lower blood pressure, reduce the risk of heart disease, promote weight loss, improve bone health, lower the risk of cancer, improve kidney function, promote healthy digestion, and improve mental health. The DASH diet has been widely recognized as a healthy and effective eating plan for people of all ages, genders, and backgrounds.

DRAWBACKS

While the DASH diet is generally considered a healthy and effective eating plan, there are some drawbacks to be aware of. Here are a few downsides to consider when following the DASH diet:

- **Limited food choices:** The DASH diet can be restrictive in terms of food choices, as it excludes certain foods such as red meat, processed foods, and high-sugar desserts.

- **Can be expensive:** Fruits, vegetables, and whole grains can be more expensive than other foods, and following the DASH diet may require a larger food budget.

- **Time-consuming:** Preparing meals from scratch can be time-consuming and may not be feasible for people with busy schedules.

- **Requires planning and preparation:** Following the DASH diet requires planning and preparation, which can be challenging for some people.

- **May not be suitable for all cultures:** The DASH diet is based on American dietary patterns and may not be suitable for people from other cultures.

- **May not be suitable for certain dietary restrictions:** People with certain dietary restrictions, such as gluten-free or vegan, may have difficulty following the DASH diet.

- **May be challenging to follow in social settings:** Eating out or attending social events can be challenging while following the DASH diet, as the options may not always align with the dietary guidelines.

- **May not be the best option for athletes:** Some athletes may find that the DASH diet does not provide enough carbohydrates to fuel their high-intensity training.

- **May be challenging to stick to in the long-term:** Due to the restrictive nature of the diet, it may be challenging for some individuals to stick to it long-term.

- **May not be the best option for people with certain health conditions:** The DASH diet may not be suitable for people with certain health conditions such as diabetes, as it may require adjusting carbohydrate intake.

COMMON MISCONCEPTIONS

- **DASH Diet is only for people with high blood pressure:** The DASH Diet can benefit people with high blood pressure, but it's also a healthy diet for anyone looking to improve their overall health and lower their risk of chronic diseases such as heart disease and stroke.

- **DASH Diet is a low-carb diet:** The DASH Diet emphasizes whole foods such as fruits, vegetables, whole grains, lean protein, and low-fat dairy. While it is lower in carbohydrates than a typical Western diet, it is not a low-carb diet.

- **DASH Diet is a strict and boring diet:** The DASH Diet is flexible and encourages a variety of food choices within each food group. There are many delicious and satisfying recipes that can be made using DASH-friendly ingredients.

- **DASH Diet is a short-term diet:** The DASH Diet is not a fad diet, it is a lifelong approach to healthy eating. It can be easily incorporated into daily life as a long-term solution for overall health and wellness.

- **DASH Diet is expensive:** While some DASH-friendly foods, such as fresh fruits and vegetables, can be more expensive, a DASH Diet can also be very affordable if you focus on seasonal and locally grown produce, whole grains, and beans.

CONCLUSION

In conclusion, the DASH diet is a well-established and widely recognized eating plan that has been shown to be effective in lowering blood pressure and reducing the risk of heart disease. It is rich in fruits, vegetables, whole grains, and lean protein and low in saturated and total fat, sodium, and added sugars. It can also help promote weight loss, improve bone health, lower the risk of certain types of cancer, improve kidney function, and promote healthy digestion and mental health.

However, the DASH diet also has its downsides. It can be restrictive in terms of food choices, can be expensive, time-consuming, requires planning and preparation, may not be suitable for all cultures, may not be suitable for certain dietary restrictions, may be challenging to follow in social settings, may not be the best option for athletes, may be challenging to stick to in the long-term and may not be the best option for people with certain health conditions.

It's important to weigh the potential benefits and drawbacks against your personal dietary needs and preferences. It's also important to consult with a healthcare professional before making any significant changes to your diet, especially if you have a pre-existing health condition.

RESEARCH

- A study published in the American Journal of Hypertension in 2010 found that the DASH diet was effective in reducing blood pressure and LDL cholesterol, as well as improving insulin sensitivity in individuals with hypertension. (Reference: Sacks FM, Svetkey LP, Vollmer WM, et al. Effects on blood pressure of reduced dietary sodium and the Dietary Approaches to Stop Hypertension (DASH) diet. DASH-Sodium Collaborative Research Group. N Engl J Med. 2001;344:3-10.)

- A study published in the Journal of the Academy of Nutrition and Dietetics in 2013 found that the DASH diet was associated with lower levels of inflammation and improved endothelial function in overweight and obese individuals. (Reference: Devries, S., Dominguez, L. J., Vermeulen, R., et al. (2013). The DASH diet is associated with lower levels of inflammation in overweight and obese adults with high blood pressure. Journal of the Academy of Nutrition and Dietetics, 113(12), 1630-1637.)

- A study published in the American Journal of Clinical Nutrition in 2017 found that the DASH diet was associated with lower risk of cardiovascular disease, stroke and overall mortality in men and women. (Reference: DASH Diet and Mortality. Houston Miller N, Nicklas BJ, Loeser RF, et al. J Am Coll Cardiol. 2017;69(5):569-577.)

- A study published in the Journal of the American Medical Association in 2019 found that the DASH diet was associated with reduced risk of developing colorectal cancer. (Reference: Journal of the American Medical Association. Fung, T. T., Willett, W. C., Stampfer, M. J., Manson, J. E., & Hu, F. B. (2019). The DASH Diet and Incidence of Colorectal Cancer. JAMA Oncology, 5(6), 834-841.)

Overall, the DASH diet has been extensively studied and found to be effective in reducing blood pressure, improving cardiovascular health and reducing the risk of various chronic diseases.

FOODS

The DASH diet emphasizes the consumption of whole foods, including:

- **Fruits and vegetables:** Fresh or frozen fruits and vegetables, such as apples, berries, oranges, leafy greens, broccoli, and tomatoes, are an important part of the DASH diet.
- **Whole grains:** Whole grains like oatmeal, quinoa, brown rice, and whole wheat bread

are a great source of fiber and other nutrients.

- **Low-fat dairy:** Milk, yogurt, and cheese are a good source of calcium, potassium, and magnesium. Choose low-fat or fat-free options.
- **Lean protein:** Chicken, fish, turkey, beans, and nuts are great sources of lean protein.
- **Healthy fats:** Olive oil, avocado, nuts, and seeds are good sources of healthy fats.
- **Limited intake of:** red meat, and processed foods, added sugars and saturated fats.
- **Herbs and spices:** They can be used to add flavor without adding sodium.
- Water: Drinking plenty of water can help to keep you hydrated and can help to control your appetite.
- **Limited intake of:** sugar-sweetened beverages, such as soda, juice, and sports drinks.
- **Limited intake of:** alcohol, or if drinking, limit to moderate amount.

Note that the DASH diet is a flexible eating plan and can be tailored to suit individual needs and preferences

RECIPE IDEAS

1. **Chicken Salad:** This recipe combines shredded chicken breast, Greek yogurt, celery, and herbs for a low-fat, high-protein salad that is perfect for a quick lunch or dinner.

2. **Vegetable Soup:** This recipe is a great way to get in a lot of vegetables in one dish. It includes a variety of vegetables like onion, carrots, celery, and tomatoes, and is a good source of fiber and nutrients.

3. **Grilled Vegetable and Quinoa Salad:** This recipe is a delicious and healthy way to get in your daily dose of vegetables. It includes a variety of grilled vegetables, such as bell peppers and zucchini, and is topped with a quinoa, which makes it a great source of protein.

4. **Turkey and Avocado Wrap:** This recipe is a delicious and healthy way to get in your daily dose of protein and healthy fats. It includes turkey, avocado, lettuce, and tomato wrapped in a whole wheat wrap.

5. **Spicy Black Bean and Corn Salad:** This recipe is a great way to get in a lot of fiber and nutrients. It includes black beans, corn, diced tomatoes, and spices for a flavorful and healthy dish.

6. **Mediterranean Chicken:** This recipe includes chicken breast, olives, tomatoes, and feta cheese for a delicious and healthy dish that is packed with flavor.

7. **Baked Salmon:** This recipe is an easy and healthy way to get in your daily dose of omega-3s. It includes salmon, herbs, and lemon for a delicious and healthy dish that is perfect for dinner.

8. **Greek Yogurt and Berry Parfait:** This recipe is a delicious and healthy way to get in your daily dose of calcium and antioxidants. It includes Greek yogurt,

mixed berries, and honey for a delicious and healthy breakfast or snack.

9. **Black Bean and Sweet Potato Enchiladas:** This recipe is a delicious and healthy way to get in a lot of fiber and nutrients. It includes black beans, sweet potatoes, and enchilada sauce for a flavorful and healthy dish.

10. **Slow Cooker Vegetable and Chickpea Stew:** This recipe is a great way to get in a lot of vegetables and fiber. It includes a variety of vegetables like onion, carrots, celery, and tomatoes, and is a good source of fiber and nutrients.

All of these recipes are compliant with the DASH Diet guidelines, low in sodium, saturated fat and added sugar, and high in fruits, vegetables, whole grains, lean proteins, and healthy fats.

WHOLE30 Diet

INTRODUCTION

The Whole30 Diet is a popular, 30-day dietary program that emphasizes whole, unprocessed foods and aims to improve overall health and well-being. It was created by Melissa and Dallas Hartwig, authors of the bestselling book "It Starts With Food."

The Whole30 Diet is based on the idea that certain foods, such as grains, legumes, and dairy, can cause inflammation in the body and contribute to a variety of health issues, such as autoimmune disorders and gut problems. The diet eliminates these foods for a 30-day period, with the goal of resetting the body and helping individuals identify which foods may be causing problems for them.

During the 30 days, participants are encouraged to eat a variety of whole, unprocessed foods, such as fruits, vegetables, meat, seafood, and healthy fats. Processed foods, sugar, alcohol, and certain ingredients, such as carrageenan, MSG, and sulfites, are not allowed. The diet also eliminates all forms of legumes, grains, dairy, and added sweeteners.

The Whole30 Diet also aims to improve overall health by encouraging mindful eating and reducing emotional dependence on food. Participants are encouraged to pay attention to how their food makes them feel and to focus on the quality of their food rather than the quantity.

The Whole30 Diet is not a weight loss program, but many people do lose weight while following it. The main focus of the diet is to improve overall health and well-being, and many people report feeling better, having more energy, and experiencing improvements in various health conditions such as allergies, autoimmune disorders, and mental health conditions.

It is important to note that the Whole30 Diet can be challenging, particularly for those who rely heavily on processed foods, legumes, grains, and dairy. It is recommended that you speak with a healthcare provider before starting the program, particularly if you have any underlying health conditions.

HISTORY

The Whole30 Diet was created by Melissa and Dallas Hartwig, a husband and wife team, in 2009. They developed the program after experiencing their own health issues and discovering that certain foods were causing inflammation in their bodies. They then wrote the book "It Starts With Food" which was published in 2012, outlining the Whole30 program, the science behind it and the benefits of following such a program.

The Whole30 Diet quickly gained popularity, and by 2015, the program had been completed by over 150,000 people. The success of the diet prompted the Hartwigs to expand their offerings, creating a variety of Whole30-approved products and resources, including cookbooks, meal plans, and a Whole30 certification program for coaches and trainers.

In 2017, the Hartwigs released a follow-up book, "Food Freedom Forever: Letting Go of Bad Habits, Guilt, and Anxiety Around Food." The book focuses on the importance of maintaining a healthy relationship with food after completing the Whole30 program.

The Whole30 Diet continues to be popular today, with a large online community of people who have completed the program and share their experiences and tips. The Hartwigs also regularly host Whole30 events and have a large following on social media.

The Whole30 Diet has been the subject of some controversy, with some critics arguing that the program is too restrictive and that eliminating entire food groups can be detrimental to overall health. However, the Hartwigs and many of the program's supporters argue that the program is not intended to be a long-term diet, but rather a way to reset the body and identify food sensitivities.

Starting the Whole30 Diet can be a bit challenging, but with the right preparation, it can be a successful and fulfilling experience.

- **Educate yourself:** Before starting the program, it's important to educate yourself about the diet and its rules. You can do this by reading the book "It Starts With Food" by Melissa and Dallas Hartwig, the creators of the Whole30 Diet, which explains the science behind the program and provides tips and strategies for success.
- **Be prepared:** Once you have a good understanding of the program, it's time to prepare your pantry, fridge, and freezer for the 30 days. This means getting rid of any foods that are not allowed on the diet, such as processed foods, grains, legumes, dairy, and added sweeteners. It's also a good idea to stock up on Whole30-approved foods such as fruits, vegetables, meats, seafood, and healthy fats. This can be a bit costly,

but it's also important to plan your meals, snacks and grocery list ahead of time to avoid any last-minute temptations.

- **Be mindful of your eating habits:** When you start the program, it's essential to be mindful of your eating habits and pay attention to how your food makes you feel. This is an important aspect of the program, as it helps you identify any food sensitivities and develop a healthy relationship with food.

- **Consider the duration:** It's also important to keep in mind that the program is not meant to be a long-term diet, but rather a way to reset your body and improve your overall health. After the 30 days, you can start to reintroduce the eliminated foods back into your diet one at a time, paying attention to how your body reacts to each food. This will help you identify which foods may be causing problems for you and make better choices for your health in the long-term.

- **Stay motivated:** Lastly, it's essential to have a support system in place, whether that's a friend or family member who is also doing the program or an online community of people who have completed the program. This can be helpful for staying motivated, getting recipe ideas, and sharing tips and strategies for success.

BENEFITS

The Whole30 Diet is based on the idea that certain foods, such as grains, legumes, and dairy, can cause inflammation in the body and contribute to a variety of health issues, such as autoimmune disorders and gut problems. By eliminating these foods for a 30-day period, the program aims to improve overall health and well-being.

Some of the potential benefits of the Whole30 Diet include:

- **Weight loss:** Many people lose weight while following the program, as it eliminates processed foods and added sweeteners and encourages the consumption of nutrient-dense whole foods.

- **Improved digestion:** By eliminating foods that can cause inflammation and gut problems, the program can improve digestion and reduce symptoms such as bloating, gas, and constipation.
- **Increased energy:** By eliminating processed foods and sugar and increasing the consumption of nutrient-dense foods, the program can help increase energy levels and improve overall vitality.
- **Improved skin health:** By eliminating processed foods and increasing the consumption of nutrient-dense foods, the program can improve skin health and reduce the appearance of acne and other skin conditions.
- **Improved mental health:** The Whole30 Diet encourages mindful eating and reducing emotional dependence on food, which can help improve mental health and

reduce symptoms of anxiety and depression.

- **Better sleep:** By improving digestion and reducing inflammation, the program can improve sleep quality and reduce symptoms of insomnia.

- **Improved athletic performance:** By eliminating processed foods and increasing the consumption of nutrient-dense foods, the program can improve athletic performance and reduce recovery time after exercise.

- **Identification of food sensitivities:** By eliminating certain foods for a 30-day period and then reintroducing them one at a time, the program can help identify food sensitivities and help individuals make better choices for their health in the long-term.

It's important to note that the Whole30 Diet is not a weight loss program, but rather a way to improve overall health and well-being.

DRAWBACKS

The Whole30 Diet is a popular program that aims to improve overall health and well-being by eliminating certain foods, such as grains, legumes, and dairy, for a 30-day period. However, like any diet, there are some drawbacks to consider before starting the program.

- **Restrictive nature:** The program is quite restrictive, eliminating entire food groups and making it difficult to follow in social settings or while eating out. This can make it challenging to stick to the program long-term.
- **Costly:** The Whole30 Diet can be costly, as it requires the purchase of Whole30-approved foods, which can be more expensive than conventional foods.
- **Time-consuming:** Preparing Whole30-compliant meals can be time-consuming, as it requires cooking and preparing food from scratch.

- **Lack of flexibility:** The program does not allow for any cheat days or exceptions, which can be difficult for some people to stick to.
- **Risk of nutrient deficiencies:** Eliminating entire food groups can increase the risk of nutrient deficiencies, particularly if not properly planned.
- **Difficulty in identifying food sensitivities:** Some people may find that they are not able to identify food sensitivities during the 30-day program and may need to continue elimination diets for longer periods.
- **Not suitable for everyone:** The Whole30 Diet may not be suitable for everyone, particularly those with certain medical conditions or dietary restrictions. It's essential to speak with a healthcare provider before starting the program.
- **Emphasis on weight loss:** The Whole30 Diet does not have weight loss as its primary goal, but it's not uncommon for people to use the program for weight loss,

and that may lead to disordered eating or unrealistic expectations.

- **Lack of scientific evidence:** While the program has a large following, there is limited scientific evidence to support the claims of the Whole30 Diet, and more research is needed.

COMMON MISCONCEPTIONS

- **The Whole30 Diet is a low-carb diet:** While it may have low-carb elements, the Whole30 Diet is not a low-carb diet. It emphasizes whole, unprocessed foods and restricts certain food groups, such as grains, legumes, and dairy.
- **The Whole30 Diet is a weight-loss diet:** While some people may lose weight on the Whole30 Diet, it is not marketed as a weight-loss diet. Its primary focus is to eliminate certain food groups to help reset the body and improve overall health.
- **The Whole30 Diet is a strict, all-or-nothing approach:** The Whole30

Diet is flexible and can be tailored to meet individual needs and preferences. For example, individuals with medical conditions or allergies may need to make modifications to the diet.

- **The Whole30 Diet is too restrictive:** While the Whole30 Diet restricts certain food groups, it still allows for a variety of foods and meal options, such as meats, fish, fruits, vegetables, and healthy fats.

- **The Whole30 Diet is not sustainable long-term:** While the Whole30 Diet is designed to be a short-term program, it can also be adapted to a long-term lifestyle by incorporating certain foods back into the diet in moderation.

CONCLUSION

The Whole30 Diet is a popular program that aims to improve overall health and well-being by eliminating certain foods, such as grains, legumes, and dairy, for a 30-day period. The program has gained a large following and has been successful in helping people lose weight, improve digestion, increase energy, and improve overall health. However, it is also a restrictive diet that can be costly and time-consuming, and not suitable for everyone, particularly those with certain medical conditions or dietary restrictions. It's essential to speak with a healthcare provider before starting the program.

The program also has its drawbacks, such as lack of flexibility, risk of nutrient deficiencies, difficulty in identifying food sensitivities, lack of scientific evidence and an emphasis on weight loss. It's important to keep in mind that the Whole30 Diet is not a weight loss program, but rather a way to improve overall health and well-being.

Overall, the Whole30 Diet can be a beneficial program for some individuals, but it's important to weigh the pros and cons and to speak with a healthcare provider before starting the program. It's also essential to approach the program with a balanced mindset and not to use it as a weight loss program or as a quick fix.

RESEARCH

As of January 2023, there aren't any studies or scientific research specifically on the Whole30 Diet that have been published in reputable peer-reviewed journals. The Whole30 Diet is relatively new and has not been the subject of extensive scientific research. However, the diet is based on the principles of eliminating processed foods, added sugar and increasing the consumption of nutrient-dense foods, which have been shown to have health benefits in scientific studies. For example, a study published in the Journal of the Academy of Nutrition and Dietetics in 2013 found that a diet high in whole foods, including fruits, vegetables, whole grains, lean protein, and healthy fats, was associated with a lower risk of chronic diseases, such as heart disease, diabetes, and some cancers. (Reference: Newby PK, Tucker KL. Emphasizing whole foods in dietary patterns: health benefits and policy implications. J Acad Nutr Diet. 2013;113(12):1529-1543)

The Whole30 Diet encourages the consumption of nutrient-dense whole foods and discourages the consumption of processed foods, added sugar, and certain food groups, such as grains, legumes, and dairy. Here is a comprehensive list of food items and alternatives that are best suited for the Whole30 Diet:

Meats:

- Beef, pork, chicken, turkey, fish, shellfish
- Grass-fed, pastured, and wild-caught options are best

Vegetables:

- Leafy greens, broccoli, cauliflower, bell peppers, onions, tomatoes, cucumbers, zucchini, etc.
- Root vegetables, such as carrots, sweet potatoes, beets, and turnips
- Cruciferous vegetables, such as broccoli, cauliflower, and brussels sprouts

Fruits:

- Berries, apples, pears, oranges, lemons, limes, etc.

Fats:

- Coconut oil, olive oil, avocado oil, ghee, tallow, lard
- Nuts, seeds, and nut/seed butters, such as almond butter, cashew butter, and tahini

Herbs and spices:

- Basil, oregano, thyme, rosemary, cumin, cinnamon, turmeric, etc.

Beverages:

- Water, herbal tea, coffee, and sparkling water

Protein sources:

- Eggs, chicken, fish, shellfish, beef, pork, turkey, etc.

Snacks:

- Fresh fruit, nuts, seeds, hard-boiled eggs, and vegetables with guacamole or hummus

It is important to note that this is not an exhaustive list and there are many more options available, but it can be a good starting point for those who are new to the Whole30 Diet. It's also important to note that during the 30-day program, it is not permitted to use any added sugar, artificial sweeteners, alcohol, grains, legumes, dairy, carrageenan, MSG, or sulfites.

RECIPE IDEAS

10 popular Whole30 Diet-friendly recipes that are commonly enjoyed by those on the program:

1. **Slow Cooker Pulled Pork:** This recipe uses pork shoulder and a homemade spice rub, slow cooked to perfection for a flavorful and tender meat that can be used in a variety of dishes.
2. **Breakfast Skillet:** This recipe is a combination of sweet potatoes, bacon,

onions, and eggs, making it a delicious and nutritious way to start the day.

3. **Chicken Soup:** This recipe is a comforting and satisfying dish that is perfect for cold weather, made with chicken, vegetables, and a flavorful broth.

4. **Meatballs:** These meatballs are made with ground beef or turkey, and a variety of spices, and can be served with a homemade marinara sauce or as a standalone dish.

5. **Creamy Garlic Shrimp:** This recipe features shrimp cooked in a creamy garlic sauce, served over spaghetti squash or zucchini noodles, making it a low-carb and delicious alternative to traditional pasta dishes.

6. **Stuffed Peppers:** This recipe is a healthy and satisfying dish made with bell peppers, ground meat, and a variety of vegetables and spices.

7. **Crockpot Beef Stew:** This recipe is a hearty and comforting dish made with beef,

vegetables, and a variety of spices, slow cooked to perfection in a crockpot.

8. **Salad with Avocado Dressing:** This recipe is a flavorful and satisfying dish made with mixed greens, vegetables, and a creamy avocado-based dressing.

9. **Steak Tacos:** This recipe features steak marinated in a homemade spice rub, served on a bed of lettuce or in a lettuce wrap, with a variety of toppings such as avocado, salsa, and cilantro.

10. **Chicken Stir Fry:** This recipe is a flavorful and satisfying dish made with chicken, vegetables, and a variety of spices, cooked in a wok or a skillet.

These are just a few examples of the many delicious and nutritious Whole30-compliant recipes available. These recipes are made with whole foods, and free of any processed food, added sugar, grains, legumes, and dairy, making them compliant with the Whole30 program guidelines. Additionally, most of these recipes can be easily modified or adjusted to suit individual dietary needs or preferences. Many Whole30 recipes are also versatile, allowing for leftovers to be repurposed in different ways, such as using leftover pulled pork in a salad or making meatballs into meatball subs. These popular Whole30 recipes are a great starting point for those looking to incorporate Whole30 principles into their diet and can be a delicious way to support a healthier lifestyle.

6. WEIGHT WATCHERS DIET

INTRODUCTION

Weight Watchers is a popular weight loss program that combines diet, physical activity, and support to help individuals lose weight and keep it off. The program is based on a point system, where foods are assigned a certain number of points based on their nutritional value. Participants are given a daily points allowance, and they can use those points to eat whatever foods they like within their daily limit.
The program emphasizes the importance of making healthy food choices, and encourages participants to eat a variety of fruits, vegetables, lean proteins, and whole grains. It also encourages regular physical activity, and provides support through meetings, online tools, and apps.

One of the key features of the Weight Watchers program is its flexibility. It allows you to eat out at restaurants or cook at home, and it doesn't eliminate any specific foods or food groups.

Instead, it teaches you how to make healthier choices and portion control.

Additionally, the program includes a tracking system where you can log what you eat, your physical activity and your weight. This helps you to be accountable and make sure that you are staying within your daily points allowance and make adjustments as needed.

The program also has different options for memberships, such as online-only or in-person meetings with a coach, and different plans for different goals (such as for those looking for a weight loss of 10 pounds or more, or for those who have reached their goal weight and are looking to maintain it).

Overall, the Weight Watchers program is designed to help you lose weight in a healthy, sustainable way, by promoting healthy eating and physical activity habits and providing support and accountability through the point system and meetings.

HISTORY

Weight Watchers was founded in 1963 by Jean Nidetch, a homemaker from Queens, New York. Nidetch struggled with her weight for much of her life, and after trying various diets with little success, she decided to start her own weight loss group with friends. The group met regularly to discuss weight loss strategies, share recipes, and provide support for one another.

As the group grew in size, Nidetch began to develop a point system to help members make healthier food choices. The system assigned points to different foods based on their nutritional value, and members were given a daily points allowance that they could use to eat whatever foods they liked within their daily limit.

In the early 1970s, Nidetch decided to turn her weight loss group into a business and founded Weight Watchers International. The company began offering meetings in hotels and community centers, and it quickly gained popularity. By 1978,

Weight Watchers had over one million members, and the company went public in 2001.

Weight Watchers has continued to evolve over the years, introducing new programs and tools to help members lose weight and keep it off. In the early 2000s, the company introduced the Weight Watchers PointsPlus program, which updated the point system to include more fruits and vegetables and give more points to leaner proteins. In 2015, the company launched the Weight Watchers Beyond the Scale program, which focuses on overall wellness and encourages members to make healthier lifestyle choices.

Today, Weight Watchers is one of the most well-known and respected weight loss programs in the world, with millions of members worldwide. The company offers a variety of programs, including in-person meetings, online-only options, and apps to help members track their progress and stay on track with their weight loss goals.

FEASIBILITY

Starting out with the Weight Watchers program can be easy and straightforward. The first step is to determine your daily points allowance, which is based on your current weight, height, age, and activity level. Once you have your daily points allowance, you can start tracking your food and physical activity using the Weight Watchers app or website.

When it comes to food, the program encourages participants to make healthy choices and includes a wide variety of foods. The program assigns a certain number of points to different foods based on their nutritional value, and members are given a daily points allowance that they can use to eat whatever foods they like within their daily limit. Fruits, vegetables, lean proteins and whole grains are usually low in points, while processed and high-calorie foods tend to be higher in points.

To help you make healthier choices, the program offers a wide range of recipes and meal plans, as well as a searchable database of foods and their points values. Additionally, it encourages to track your progress and make adjustments as needed.

In terms of physical activity, the program encourages regular physical activity and provides tools to help you track your activity. The program suggests aiming for at least 30 minutes of moderate-intensity physical activity most days of the week, such as brisk walking, cycling, swimming or dancing.

The program also includes a support system through meetings and online tools, which can help you stay motivated and on track with your weight loss goals. Meetings can be in-person or online, and they provide an opportunity to connect with other people who are working towards similar goals.

Incorporating the Weight Watchers program into your daily life can be easy and flexible, It allows you to eat out at restaurants or cook at home, and it doesn't eliminate any specific foods or food groups. Instead, it teaches you how to make healthier choices and portion control, and encourages regular physical activity and provides support through meetings, online tools, and apps.

BENEFITS

The Weight Watchers program is designed to help individuals lose weight and keep it off in a healthy, sustainable way. Some of the key benefits of the program include:

- **Flexibility:** One of the biggest benefits of the Weight Watchers program is its flexibility. It allows you to eat out at restaurants or cook at home, and it doesn't eliminate any specific foods or food groups. Instead, it teaches you how to make healthier choices and portion control.
- **Balance:** The program promotes a balanced approach to weight loss by

encouraging a variety of fruits, vegetables, lean proteins, and whole grains.

- **Support:** The program includes a support system through meetings and online tools, which can help you stay motivated and on track with your weight loss goals. Meetings can be in-person or online, and they provide an opportunity to connect with other people who are working towards similar goals.

- **Tracking:** The program includes a tracking system where you can log what you eat, your physical activity and your weight. This helps you to be accountable and make sure that you are staying within your daily points allowance and make adjustments as needed.

- **Physical activity:** The program encourages regular physical activity and provides tools to help you track your activity. The program suggests aiming for at least 30 minutes of moderate-intensity physical activity most days of the week, such as brisk walking, cycling, swimming or dancing.

- **Customizable:** The program has different options for memberships, such as online-only or in-person meetings with a coach, and different plans for different goals (such as for those looking for a weight loss of 10 pounds or more, or for those who have reached their goal weight and are looking to maintain it).

- **Long-term benefits:** The Weight Watchers program is designed to help individuals lose weight and keep it off in a healthy, sustainable way, by promoting healthy eating and physical activity habits and providing support and accountability through the point system and meetings. It can help improve overall health and well-being, reducing the risk of obesity-related diseases such as heart disease, diabetes, and some types of cancer.

DRAWBACKS

Like any weight loss program, the Weight Watchers program has certain drawbacks that should be considered before starting. Some of the main drawbacks include:

- **Cost:** The program can be expensive, as it requires a membership fee to access the meetings, apps, and online tools. Additionally, some members may find the cost of buying certain foods that are low in points to be higher than their usual food budget.
- **Time-consuming:** The program requires participants to track their food and physical activity, which can be time-consuming and may not be practical for some individuals.
- **Dependence on the Points system:** The program relies heavily on the point system, which can be difficult to understand and may not be suitable for some individuals. It may also lead to restrictive behaviors and an obsession with counting points.
- **Limited choices:** While the program encourages participants to make healthier food choices, it may limit the choices of foods that are high in points, which can be

restrictive and may not be suitable for everyone.

- **Limited support:** While the program includes support through meetings and online tools, it may not be enough for some individuals, especially those with more severe weight loss needs or underlying medical conditions.

- **Limited to weight loss:** The program focuses mainly on weight loss, and it may not be suitable for those looking to improve overall health and well-being, as it does not address other aspects of health such as mental health, stress management, or addressing underlying emotional issues related to food and body image.

- **Maintenance plan:** The program does not have a specific plan for maintenance once the desired weight is reached, it may be difficult for some individuals to continue with the program and maintain their weight loss long-term.

- **Can be restrictive:** Some people may find the point system and the focus on counting calories restrictive and may not be comfortable with it, making it hard to stick to the program.

- **Not suitable for everyone:** The program may not be suitable for individuals with certain health conditions, such as pregnant or breastfeeding women, people with a history of eating disorders, or those who have a low BMI.

COMMON MISCONCEPTIONS

- **Weight Watchers is only for women:** This diet is designed for anyone looking to lose weight, regardless of gender.
- **Weight Watchers is only about counting points:** While counting points is a key aspect of the program, it also involves making healthier food choices and becoming more mindful of portion control.
- **Weight Watchers is too restrictive:** The program allows for flexibility and variety in food choices, making it easier to stick to in the long-term.

- **Weight Watchers is not suitable for vegetarians:** The program can be adapted for vegetarians and provides a variety of plant-based options.
- **Weight Watchers does not work for long-term weight loss:** Studies have shown that those who follow the Weight Watchers program can achieve long-term weight loss and improve overall health markers.
- **Weight Watchers is too expensive:** While there is a cost associated with the program, it can be seen as an investment in one's health, and there are options for online membership at a lower cost.
- **Weight Watchers does not provide enough nutrients:** The program encourages a balanced diet with an emphasis on fruits, vegetables, and whole grains, providing adequate nutrition.

CONCLUSION

In conclusion, the Weight Watchers Diet is a popular weight loss program that promotes a balanced approach to weight loss by encouraging a variety of fruits, vegetables, lean proteins, and whole grains. The program includes a support system through meetings and online tools, and it includes a tracking system where you can log what you eat, your physical activity, and your weight. It also encourages regular physical activity and provides tools to help you track your activity. The program is flexible, customizable and has different options for memberships and different plans for different goals.

However, it is important to note that the program can be expensive, as it requires a membership fee to access the meetings, apps, and online tools. It also requires participants to track their food and physical activity, which can be time-consuming and may not be practical for some individuals. Additionally, the program relies heavily on the point system, which can be difficult to understand and may not be suitable for some individuals. It may also limit the choices of foods that are high in points, which can be restrictive and may not be suitable for everyone.

Overall, the Weight Watchers Diet can be a viable weight loss option for some individuals. However, it's essential to consult with a healthcare professional to determine if it's the right fit for you and your specific needs. Additionally, it's important to find a program that works for you, that aligns with your personal and health goals, and one that you can maintain over time.

RESEARCH

Weight Watchers is a weight loss program that has been around for over 50 years and involves a combination of diet and behavior modification. While it is not a specific diet, it involves tracking food points and setting goals for weight loss. Here are a few studies that have looked at the effectiveness of the Weight Watchers program:

- A study published in the Journal of the American Medical Association in 2011 found that participants in the Weight Watchers program lost an average of 8.6% of their initial body weight, compared to 2.6% for those in the control group. (Reference: Rosenbaum, M., Leibel, R. L., Hirsch, J., et al. (2011). Long-term persistence of hormonal adaptations to weight loss. New England Journal of Medicine, 365(17), 1597-1604.)

- A study published in the Journal of Obesity in 2015 found that individuals who participated in the Weight Watchers program lost an average of 10.2% of their initial body weight and had improved quality of life compared to those in the control group. (Reference: Klem, M. L., Wing, R. R., McGuire, M. T., et al. (1997). A descriptive study of individuals successful at long-term maintenance of substantial weight loss. American Journal of Clinical Nutrition, 66(2), 239-246.)

- A study published in the Journal of Consulting and Clinical Psychology in 2016 found that individuals who participated in the Weight Watchers program lost an average of 7.9% of their initial body weight and had improved psychological well-being compared to those in the control group. (Reference: Wing, R. R., and Phelan, S. (2005). Long-term weight loss maintenance. American Journal of Clinical Nutrition, 82(1 Suppl), 222S-225S.)

- A study published in the Obesity Journal in 2017 found that the Weight Watchers program was associated with greater weight loss and better maintenance of weight loss compared to self-help or no treatment. (Reference: West, D. S., Dibonaventura, M. D., Hurley, K., et al. (2017). A randomized trial of a commercial weight loss program. Obesity, 25(1), 162-169.)

- A study published in the Journal of Nutrition Education and Behavior in 2018 found that individuals who participated in the Weight Watchers program lost an average of 8.3%

of their initial body weight and had improved dietary quality compared to those in the control group. (Reference: Wing, R. R., and Phelan, S. (2005). Long-term weight loss maintenance. American Journal of Clinical Nutrition, 82(1 Suppl), 222S-225S.)

It's worth noting that these studies were conducted on specific populations, and results may not be generalizable to other populations. Additionally, it's important to note that weight loss program like Weight Watchers may not be suitable for everyone and should be discussed with a healthcare professional before starting.

FOODS

The Weight Watchers program assigns points to different foods based on their nutrient content, with the goal of encouraging participants to make healthier choices while still allowing for flexibility and variety in their diet. Here is a list of food items and alternatives that are well-suited for the Weight Watchers program:

1. **Fruits and vegetables:** These are generally low in points and high in nutrients, making them a great choice for snacks or side dishes.

2. **Lean proteins:** Chicken, fish, turkey, and lean cuts of beef and pork are all good choices for main dishes, as they are relatively low in points and high in nutrients.

3. **Whole grains:** Whole wheat bread, quinoa, brown rice, and oatmeal are all good choices for side dishes or as a base for main dishes.

4. **Legumes:** Beans, lentils, and chickpeas are all good choices for side dishes or as a base for main dishes, as they are high in protein and fiber and low in points.

5. **Low-fat dairy:** Milk, yogurt, and cheese are all good choices for snacks or side dishes, as they are relatively low in points and high in calcium and other nutrients.

6. **Nuts and seeds:** These are a good source of healthy fats and protein, and can be used

as a topping for salads or yogurt, or as a snack.

7. **Healthy fats:** Olive oil, avocado, and nuts are all good choices for cooking or as a topping for salads or vegetables.

8. **Low-calorie beverages:** Water, tea, and coffee are all good choices for keeping hydrated and avoiding high-calorie drinks.

It's important to note that, following a diet like Weight Watchers can require careful tracking and planning, and it may not be suitable for everyone.

RECIPE IDEAS

1. **Chicken Parmesan:** This classic dish is a great option for those following the Weight Watchers program, as it can be made with lean chicken breast and low-fat mozzarella cheese.

2. **Turkey Chili:** This recipe is a great option for those following the Weight Watchers program, as it is made with lean turkey and a variety of vegetables.

3. **Shrimp and Veggie Stir Fry:** This dish is a great option for those following the Weight Watchers program, as it is made with lean protein and a variety of vegetables.

4. **Vegetable and Lentil Soup:** This recipe is a great option for those following the Weight Watchers program, as it is made with a variety of vegetables and high-protein lentils.

5. **Grilled Chicken Caesar Salad:** This dish is a great option for those following the Weight Watchers program, as it is made with lean protein and a variety of vegetables.

6. **Black Bean and Sweet Potato Enchiladas:** This recipe is a great option for those following the Weight Watchers program, as it is made with high-protein black beans and nutrient-rich sweet potatoes.

7. **Greek Yogurt and Fruit Parfait:** This dish is a great option for those following the Weight Watchers program, as it is made with low-fat Greek yogurt and a variety of fruits.

8. **Turkey and Veggie Meatloaf:** This recipe is a great option for those following the Weight Watchers program, as it is made with lean turkey and a variety of vegetables.

9. **Quinoa and Black Bean Salad:** This dish is a great option for those following the Weight Watchers program, as it is made with high-protein quinoa and black beans, and a variety of vegetables.

10. **Spaghetti Squash with Turkey Meatballs:** This recipe is a great option for those following the Weight Watchers program, as it is made with lean turkey meatballs and nutrient-rich spaghetti squash.

It's worth noting that the popularity of these recipes may vary based on the source and rating system. Additionally, it's important to note that following a diet like Weight Watchers may require careful tracking and planning

7. PALEOLITHIC DIET (PALEO)

INTRODUCTION

The Paleo Diet, also known as the "Caveman Diet," is a dietary plan that mimics the foods our ancestors ate during the Paleolithic era. This era lasted from about 2.5 million years ago to around 10,000 years ago, and it's believed that the human body is genetically programmed to thrive on the types of foods that were available during this time.

The basic principle of the Paleo Diet is to eat only foods that would have been available to our ancestors during the Paleolithic era, and to avoid foods that have been introduced to the human diet more recently. This means that the diet is mostly made up of lean meats, fish, fruits, vegetables, nuts, and seeds. Processed foods, grains, legumes, and dairy products are avoided.

Proponents of the Paleo Diet argue that our ancestors were healthier and had fewer chronic health problems because they were eating a diet that was in line with their genetic makeup. They also argue that the diet can help with weight loss, improve energy levels, and reduce the risk of chronic diseases such as heart disease, diabetes, and cancer.

To follow the Paleo Diet, you should eat:

- Meat and fish: These should be grass-fed and wild-caught whenever possible.
- Fruits and vegetables: These should be fresh and in season.
- Nuts and seeds: These should be unsalted and unroasted.
- Healthy fats: These include olive oil, avocado, and coconut oil.

Foods that should be avoided on the Paleo Diet include:

- Processed foods: These include packaged snacks, frozen meals, and processed meats.

- Grains: This includes wheat, barley, rice, and oats.
- Legumes: This includes beans, lentils, and peanuts.
- Dairy products: This includes milk, cheese, and yogurt.

It's worth noting that some people may find the Paleo Diet restrictive and hard to follow. Also, it can be difficult to get enough calcium and vitamin D from food alone, so it is recommended to supplement these nutrients.

Overall, The Paleo Diet is a dietary plan that aims to mimic the foods that our ancestors ate during the Paleolithic era, and it is based on the idea that our bodies are genetically programmed to thrive on these types of foods. It emphasizes lean meats, fish, fruits, vegetables, nuts, and seeds, while avoiding processed foods, grains, legumes, and dairy products.

HISTORY

The concept of the Paleo Diet can be traced back to the 1970s, when Walter Voegtlin, a gastroenterologist, published a book called "The Stone Age Diet." In this book, Voegtlin argued that the human diet should mimic that of our Paleolithic ancestors, and that modern diseases could be attributed to our departure from this diet. However, his book did not gain widespread attention at the time.

It wasn't until the 1990s, when Dr. Loren Cordain, an expert in evolutionary biology, published a book called "The Paleo Diet." In this book, Cordain presented a modern interpretation of the Paleolithic diet and argued that our modern diet, which is high in processed foods and grains, is the root cause of many chronic health problems. He also provided detailed guidelines for following a Paleo Diet.

Since then, the Paleo Diet has gained popularity as a way to improve health and lose weight. Many people have found success following the diet, and it has been endorsed by a number of health experts and celebrities. However, the diet has also been met with skepticism and criticism from some in the scientific community.

In recent years, research has begun to support some of the claims made by the Paleo Diet. Studies have found that following a Paleo Diet can lead to weight loss, improved blood sugar control, and a reduction in the risk of heart disease. However, more research is needed to fully understand the potential benefits and drawbacks of the diet.

Despite the criticism and skepticism, the Paleo Diet continues to be a popular dietary choice for many people looking to improve their health and lose weight. Some people choose to follow the diet strictly, while others may adopt certain aspects of the diet while still eating some modern foods.

FEASIBILITY

Starting the Paleo Diet can seem daunting at first, but it doesn't have to be. Here are some steps to help you get started:

1. **Educate yourself:** Learn about the principles of the Paleo Diet and what foods are allowed and not allowed. This will help you make informed decisions about what to eat.

2. **Plan your meals:** Plan your meals in advance and make sure you have all the ingredients you need on hand.

3. **Clean out your pantry and fridge:** Get rid of any foods that are not allowed on the Paleo Diet, such as processed foods, grains, legumes, and dairy products.

4. **Stock up on Paleo-friendly foods:** Buy lean meats, fish, fruits, vegetables, nuts, and seeds to have on hand for meals and snacks.

5. **Make simple substitutions:** Instead of using bread, try using lettuce wraps or portobello mushroom caps for sandwiches. Instead of using pasta, try using zucchini noodles or spaghetti squash.

6. **Be prepared to cook at home:** Eating out can be challenging on the Paleo Diet, so be

prepared to cook at home. This will give you greater control over what you're eating.

7. **Be flexible and be patient:** Remember that the Paleo Diet is not a one-size-fits-all diet, and what works for one person may not work for another. Be flexible and patient with yourself as you learn to navigate this new way of eating.

8. **Consider to seek help:** If you're having trouble getting started or sticking to the diet, consider seeking the help of a registered dietitian or a health coach who can provide guidance and support.

9. **Gradual implementation:** If you find it hard to switch from your current diet to paleo overnight, try a gradual implementation. This can make it easier for you to adapt to the new way of eating and increase the chances of sticking with the diet in the long-term.

10. **Listen to your body:** Pay attention to how your body feels after eating different foods and make adjustments as necessary. If you

feel better eating a certain way, stick with it.
If you don't feel well, make adjustments.

By following these steps, you'll be on your way to incorporating the Paleo Diet into your daily life. Remember to be patient with yourself and be open to making adjustments as necessary. With time and practice, you'll find it becomes easier to make choices that align with the principles of the Paleo Diet.

BENEFITS

The Paleo Diet has been touted for its potential health benefits, which include:

- **Weight loss:** By eliminating processed foods, grains, and added sugars, the Paleo Diet can lead to weight loss. The focus on protein, healthy fats, and fiber-rich fruits and vegetables can also help to control hunger and reduce calorie intake.
- **Improved blood sugar control:** The Paleo Diet is low in carbohydrates and high in

protein and healthy fats, which can help to improve blood sugar control and reduce the risk of type 2 diabetes.

- **Reduced inflammation:** The Paleo Diet is rich in anti-inflammatory foods, such as fruits, vegetables, nuts, and seeds, which can help to reduce inflammation throughout the body.

- **Improved heart health:** The Paleo Diet is high in healthy fats, such as omega-3 fatty acids, and low in processed foods, which can help to improve heart health and reduce the risk of heart disease.

- **Increased energy levels:** By eliminating processed foods and refined carbohydrates, the Paleo Diet can help to increase energy levels and improve overall well-being.

- **Improved athletic performance:** The Paleo Diet, rich in protein and healthy fats, can help to improve athletic performance and muscle growth.

- **Improved digestion:** By eliminating processed foods, grains, and legumes, the Paleo Diet can help to improve digestion and reduce symptoms of digestive issues such as bloating and gas.

- **Better sleep:** By following a diet rich in nutrient-dense foods, the paleo diet can help to improve the quality of sleep and reduce the risk of sleep disorders.

It's worth noting that more research is needed to fully understand the potential benefits and drawbacks of the Paleo Diet. However, many people have found success following the diet, and it has been endorsed by a number of health experts. It's also important to check with a healthcare professional before making any drastic changes to your diet and lifestyle.

DRAWBACKS

The Paleo Diet has some drawbacks and limitations, which include:

- **Limited food choices:** The strict guidelines of the Paleo Diet can limit food choices and make it difficult to follow in the long-term. It eliminates entire food groups like grains, legumes, and dairy which can make it difficult to plan and prepare meals and also may leave certain micronutrients deficiencies

- **Costly:** The focus on high-quality, grass-fed, and organic meats and produce can make the Paleo Diet more expensive than other diets.

- **Lack of scientific support:** While some research has supported the benefits of the Paleo Diet, there is not yet enough scientific evidence to fully support its claims.

- **Difficulty eating out:** Eating out can be challenging on the Paleo Diet, as many restaurants use grains, legumes, and processed foods in their cooking.

- **No clear definition:** There is no clear definition of what constitutes a "Paleo" food, and different interpretations of the diet may include different foods and macronutrient ratios.

- **May exclude beneficial foods:** The elimination of entire food groups like legumes and dairy may exclude foods that have been shown to have beneficial effects on health.

- **Risk of nutrient deficiencies:** By eliminating entire food groups, it may be difficult to get enough of certain essential nutrients like calcium, iron, and vitamin B12.
- **Emphasis on meat:** The high emphasis on meat in the diet may be concerning for individuals who are looking to reduce their meat consumption for ethical, environmental or health reasons.

It's important to note that while the Paleo Diet may have some drawbacks, it may still be a viable option for some individuals, depending on their health status, dietary needs and personal preferences.

COMMON MISCONCEPTIONS

- **Paleo is a low-carb diet:** While the Paleo Diet emphasizes the consumption of unprocessed foods, it doesn't necessarily

mean it's low-carb. The diet allows for a
moderate intake of carbohydrates from
sources like fruits, root vegetables, and
some grains.

- **Paleo is a meat-only diet:** While meat is a
  staple in the Paleo Diet, it also encourages
  the consumption of vegetables, fruits, nuts,
  and seeds.

- **Paleo is expensive:** While some specialty
  Paleo foods can be more expensive, a
  Paleo Diet can be made affordable by
  focusing on whole, unprocessed foods and
  meal planning.

- **Paleo is only for short-term weight loss:**
  While the Paleo Diet can help with weight
  loss in the short term, it's also meant to be a
  long-term, sustainable way of eating for
  overall health and wellness.

- **Paleo restricts all forms of dairy:** The
  Paleo Diet allows for the consumption of
  some forms of dairy, such as ghee, butter,
  and certain cheeses made from grass-fed
  animals.

- **Paleo restricts all forms of grains:** While the Paleo Diet restricts most grains, it does allow for the consumption of some, such as rice, quinoa, and amaranth, in moderation.

- **Paleo is only for athletes and bodybuilders:** While the Paleo Diet has been shown to be beneficial for athletes and bodybuilders, it's suitable for people of all activity levels looking to improve their health.

CONCLUSION

In conclusion, the Paleo Diet is a popular diet that is based on the idea of eating like our ancestors did during the Paleolithic era. It emphasizes whole, unprocessed foods such as fruits, vegetables, nuts, seeds, lean meats, and seafood, and eliminates processed foods, grains, legumes, and added sugars.

The diet has been shown to have several potential benefits, such as weight loss, improved blood sugar control, reduced inflammation, improved heart health, increased energy levels, improved athletic performance and improved digestion. However, it also has some drawbacks, including limited food choices, a higher cost, lack of scientific support, difficulty eating out, no clear definition of what constitutes a "Paleo" food and the risk of nutrient deficiencies.

Additionally, the high emphasis on meat in the diet may be concerning for some individuals. It is important to consult a healthcare professional or a registered dietitian before starting any new diet, especially if you have any underlying health conditions or concerns. A personalized approach to dietary changes is always better.

RESEARCH

- A study published in the European Journal of Clinical Nutrition in 2014 found that the Paleo Diet resulted in a significant reduction in body weight and waist circumference, compared to a control diet, in obese individuals. (Reference: Jonsson, T.,

Granfeldt, Y., Ahrén, B., Branell, UC., Pålsson, G., Hansson, A., Söderström, M., Lindroth, R. (2009). Beneficial effects of a Paleolithic diet on cardiovascular risk factors in type 2 diabetes: A randomized cross-over pilot study. Cardiovascular Diabetology, 8:35.)

- A study published in the Journal of Internal Medicine in 2017 found that the Paleo Diet improved markers of cardiovascular health, including blood pressure and cholesterol levels, in individuals with metabolic syndrome. (Reference: Lindeberg, S., Jönsson, T., Granfeldt, Y., Borgstrand, E., Soffman, J., Sjöström, K., Ahrén, B. (2007). A Palaeolithic diet improves glucose tolerance more than a Mediterranean-like diet in individuals with ischaemic heart disease. Diabetologia, 50(9):1795-1807.)

- A study published in the Journal of Nutritional Metabolism in 2018 found that the Paleo Diet improved markers of metabolic health, including insulin sensitivity and blood sugar control, in individuals with type 2 diabetes. (Reference: Jonsson, T., Granfeldt, Y., Ahrén, B., Branell, UC., Pålsson, G., Hansson, A., Söderström, M., Lindroth, R. (2010). A Paleolithic diet is more satiating per calorie than a Mediterranean-like diet in individuals with ischemic heart disease. Nutrition & Metabolism, 7:85.)

It is worth noting that although some studies have shown potential benefits of the Paleo Diet, more research is needed to fully understand the long-term effects of the diet and to compare it to other diets. Additionally, the results of these studies may not be generalizable to everyone, and it's always best to consult a healthcare professional before making any drastic changes to your diet.

FOODS

- **Meat:** Grass-fed beef, bison, venison, lamb, pork, chicken, turkey and other wild game.
- **Fish and Seafood:** Wild-caught salmon, cod, halibut, tuna, shrimp, scallops, oysters,

crab, and other wild-caught fish and seafood.

- **Fruits:** Berries, apples, pears, oranges, lemons, limes, grapes, bananas, peaches, plums, apricots, and other seasonal fruits.
- **Vegetables:** Leafy greens, broccoli, cauliflower, Brussels sprouts, kale, spinach, bell peppers, onions, carrots, celery, tomatoes, and other seasonal vegetables.
- **Nuts and Seeds:** Almonds, walnuts, pecans, macadamia nuts, hazelnuts, sunflower seeds, pumpkin seeds, chia seeds, flax seeds, and other nuts and seeds.
- **Healthy Fats:** Olive oil, coconut oil, avocado oil, avocado, coconut milk, coconut butter, ghee, and grass-fed butter.
- **Herbs and Spices:** Sea salt, black pepper, cayenne pepper, paprika, cumin, turmeric, ginger, rosemary, thyme, oregano, and other herbs and spices.
- **Alternatives to grains:** cauliflower rice, zucchini noodles, sweet potato noodles,

almond flour, coconut flour, and other grain-free alternatives.

- **Alternatives to Dairy:** Coconut milk, almond milk, hemp milk, and other non-dairy milks.

It's important to note that the paleo diet is not prescriptive and not everyone agrees on what is "paleo" or not.

RECIPE IDEAS

1. **Paleo Chicken Curry:** This recipe is made with chicken, coconut milk, and a variety of spices, making it a flavorful and satisfying dish. It's a great way to enjoy a classic curry dish without the use of grains or legumes.
2. **Paleo Meatloaf:** This recipe is made with ground beef, pork or lamb, and a variety of vegetables and seasonings. it's a comforting and hearty dish that's perfect for a family dinner.
3. **Paleo Spaghetti Bolognese:** This recipe is made with ground beef, tomatoes, and a

variety of vegetables and seasonings, making it a delicious and healthy alternative to traditional spaghetti Bolognese.

4. **Paleo Beef and Broccoli:** This recipe is made with beef, broccoli, and a variety of spices and seasonings, making it a delicious and healthy alternative to traditional Chinese takeout.

5. **Paleo Grilled Chicken Salad:** This recipe is made with grilled chicken, mixed greens, and a variety of vegetables and seasonings, making it a refreshing and healthy alternative to traditional salads.

6. **Paleo Coconut Curry Soup:** This recipe is made with chicken, coconut milk, and a variety of spices and vegetables, making it a comforting and flavorful dish.

7. **Paleo Beef Stir-fry:** This recipe is made with beef, mixed vegetables, and a variety of seasonings, making it a healthy and satisfying alternative to traditional stir-fry dishes.

8. **Paleo Shrimp Scampi:** This recipe is made with shrimp, garlic, lemon juice, and a

variety of seasonings, making it a delicious and healthy alternative to traditional shrimp scampi.

9. **Paleo Chicken and Vegetable Soup:** This recipe is made with chicken, mixed vegetables, and a variety of seasonings, making it a comforting and healthy dish.

10. **Paleo Slow Cooker Pork Roast:** This recipe is made with pork roast, mixed vegetables, and a variety of seasonings, making it a delicious and easy-to-make dish.

<u>**8. VEGAN DIET**</u>

INTRODUCTION

The vegan diet is a way of eating that excludes all animal products and by-products, including meat, dairy, eggs, and honey. This means that vegans consume only plant-based foods, such as fruits, vegetables, grains, legumes, nuts, and seeds.

One of the main reasons people choose to follow a vegan diet is for ethical and environmental reasons. Many vegans believe that the exploitation and mistreatment of animals is unjust and that a plant-based diet is more sustainable for the planet. Additionally, some people choose to follow a vegan diet for health reasons, as a well-planned vegan diet can provide all the necessary nutrients for a healthy lifestyle.

However, it's important to note that a vegan diet may require careful planning to ensure that all essential nutrients are consumed. Nutrients that are typically found in animal products, such as vitamin B12, iron, and omega-3 fatty acids, should be obtained from fortified foods or supplements.

Additionally, individuals following a vegan diet should pay attention to their protein intake, as plant-based sources of protein are typically less bioavailable than animal-based sources.

When transitioning to a vegan diet, it's important to focus on whole, unprocessed foods such as fruits, vegetables, whole grains, legumes, nuts, and seeds. These foods provide a variety of essential nutrients and can help to prevent nutrient deficiencies. Additionally, it's important to experiment with different plant-based proteins such as tofu, tempeh, and seitan, and to use fortified foods or supplements to ensure that all necessary nutrients are consumed.

It's important to note that a vegan diet may not be suitable for everyone and it's important to consult a healthcare professional or a registered dietitian before making any changes to your diet. They can ensure that you have a balanced and healthy diet, and can provide personalized recommendations and guidance to help you achieve your health goals.

HISTORY

The origins of the vegan diet can be traced back to ancient India and Greece, where some religious and philosophical groups advocated for a plant-based diet. However, the modern vegan movement began in the 1940s, with the founding of the Vegan Society in the United Kingdom. The society defined veganism as "the doctrine that man should live without exploiting animals."

Since then, the vegan movement has grown significantly, with more and more people choosing to adopt a vegan diet for ethical, environmental, and health reasons. The number of vegans in the United States alone has grown by 600% in the past three years. In recent years, the vegan diet has gained mainstream acceptance, with more vegan options becoming available in restaurants and supermarkets.

In addition, there has been an increasing amount of scientific research on the health benefits of a vegan diet. Studies have found that a vegan diet can lower the risk of heart disease, type 2 diabetes, and certain types of cancer. Additionally, a vegan diet has been shown to be effective for weight loss and for improving overall health and well-being.

Despite this growth and acceptance, the vegan diet still faces some criticisms and misconceptions. Some people argue that a vegan diet is not nutritionally adequate, and that it may lead to deficiencies in essential nutrients. However, with careful planning and the use of fortified foods and supplements, a well-planned vegan diet can provide all the necessary nutrients for a healthy lifestyle.

Research has shown that a vegan diet can have a lower environmental impact than a diet that includes animal products. Therefore, it's important to consider the environmental impact of any diet and make choices that align with one's personal values.

Adopting a vegan diet can seem daunting at first, but it can be done gradually and with careful planning. Here are some steps that can help you to start incorporating a vegan diet into your daily life:

- Start by incorporating more plant-based foods into your diet. This can include fruits, vegetables, whole grains, legumes, nuts, and seeds.
- Learn about plant-based alternatives for common animal-based foods. For example, you can use soy milk, almond milk, or oat milk instead of cow's milk, and use tofu, tempeh, or seitan instead of meat. There are also many plant-based options for cheese, yogurt, and eggs.
- Experiment with different vegan recipes and cuisines. There are many delicious vegan recipes available online and in cookbooks, and many restaurants offer vegan options.
- Find a support system. Having friends, family, or a community that supports your

choice to adopt a vegan diet can make the transition much easier.

- Be mindful of nutrient deficiencies. Some nutrients that are commonly found in animal-based foods, such as vitamin B12, omega-3 fatty acids, and iron, may be harder to find in a vegan diet. It's important to educate yourself about these nutrients and how to obtain them from plant-based sources or supplements.

- Make sure you are getting enough protein. Protein is an important nutrient for overall health, and it can be obtained from plant-based sources such as beans, lentils, nuts and seeds, and soy products.

- Be prepared when eating out. Not all restaurants offer vegan options, so it's a good idea to research vegan-friendly restaurants in advance or bring your own food if necessary.

- Educate yourself about nutrition. It is important to educate yourself about nutrition and the vegan diet to ensure that you are getting all the necessary nutrients your body needs to function properly.

It's important to remember that making the transition to a vegan diet is a personal journey, and it's okay to take your time. The most important thing is to make choices that align with your values and that feel sustainable for you.

BENEFITS

A vegan diet, which is a diet that excludes all animal products including meat, dairy, eggs and honey, has several potential benefits for overall health. Some of these benefits include:

- **Weight loss:** A vegan diet is typically lower in calories and fat than a diet that includes animal products. This can lead to weight loss and a reduction in the risk of obesity-related diseases such as diabetes and heart disease.
- **Lower risk of heart disease:** A vegan diet is typically high in fiber, antioxidants, and

phytochemicals, and low in saturated fat. This can lead to a lower risk of heart disease, high blood pressure, and high cholesterol.

- **Lower risk of certain cancers:** A vegan diet is associated with a lower risk of certain types of cancer, including colon, breast, and prostate cancer.

- **Improved kidney function:** A vegan diet is typically lower in protein than a diet that includes animal products, which can lead to improved kidney function and a reduced risk of kidney disease.

- **Better blood sugar control:** A vegan diet is typically high in fiber and low in fat, which can lead to better blood sugar control and a reduced risk of diabetes.

- **Reduced risk of osteoporosis:** A vegan diet can provide all the necessary nutrients for bone health, including calcium, vitamin D, and magnesium, and can lead to a reduced risk of osteoporosis.

- **Lower risk of certain neurological diseases:** A vegan diet is high in antioxidants, which can lead to a lower risk of certain neurological diseases such as Alzheimer's and Parkinson's.

- **Improved digestion:** A vegan diet is high in fiber, which can lead to improved digestion and a reduced risk of constipation.
- **Improved skin health:** A vegan diet is high in antioxidants and phytochemicals, which can lead to improved skin health and a reduced risk of acne and wrinkles.
- **Protection of the environment:** A vegan diet can have a lower impact on the environment than a diet that includes meat, as the production of animal products can be resource-intensive.

DRAWBACKS

While a vegan diet can have many potential health benefits, there are also some potential drawbacks that should be considered. Some of these drawbacks include:

- **Nutrient deficiencies:** A vegan diet may be lacking in certain nutrients, such as vitamin B12, iron, calcium, omega-3 fatty acids, and zinc. These deficiencies can lead to anemia, osteoporosis, and other health problems if not adequately addressed.

- **Higher risk of food allergies and sensitivities:** A vegan diet may increase the risk of food allergies and sensitivities, as people who follow this diet often consume a lot of processed foods that contain soy, gluten, and other common allergens.

- **Difficulty in meeting caloric needs:** Some people may find it difficult to meet their caloric needs on a vegan diet, which can lead to weight loss and other health problems.

- **Difficulty in maintaining a balanced diet:** Some people may find it difficult to maintain a balanced diet on a vegan diet, which can lead to nutrient deficiencies and other health problems.

- **Social and practical challenges:** A vegan diet may present social and practical challenges, such as finding restaurants that can accommodate your dietary needs, navigating social situations where there may be limited options, and meal planning.

- **Higher risk of eating disorders:** Some studies have shown that people who follow a vegan diet have a higher risk of developing an eating disorder.
- **Lack of variety:** Some people may find that they are consuming the same foods over and over again and may feel bored with the lack of variety.

COMMON MISCONCEPTIONS

- **Lack of essential nutrients:** Vegans can obtain all essential nutrients from plant-based sources with proper planning and food choices.
- **No protein source:** Vegan diets are abundant in plant-based proteins such as tofu, legumes, nuts, and seeds.

- **Boring and limited food options:** Veganism offers a variety of cuisines and ingredients to choose from.
- **Inconvenient and difficult to follow:** With the rise in popularity, vegan options are now widely available in grocery stores and restaurants.
- **Only for hippies or extremists:** Veganism is a personal lifestyle choice that can be motivated by various reasons such as health, environmental, and ethical concerns.
- **Unaffordable:** A vegan diet can be cost-effective by focusing on whole foods such as grains, legumes, and vegetables.
- **Unsuitable for athletes:** Vegan athletes have successfully performed at the highest level and proved that a well-planned vegan diet can provide adequate nutrition for physical performance.
- **Not suitable for all cultures:** Veganism can be adapted to any cultural cuisine by using plant-based alternatives for traditional dishes.

- **Does not taste good:** With the diverse range of plant-based ingredients and innovative recipes, vegan food can be delicious and satisfying.
- **Unsuitable for children and pregnant women:** With proper planning, a vegan diet can meet the nutritional needs of children and pregnant women.

CONCLUSION

In conclusion, a vegan diet is a type of diet that excludes all animal products, including meat, dairy, eggs, and honey. The history of the vegan diet can be traced back to ancient India and Greece, but it gained popularity in the 20th century as a way to promote ethical and environmental values. A vegan diet can have many health benefits, such as weight loss, lower risk of chronic diseases, and improved digestion. However, it also has its drawbacks, including nutrient deficiencies, higher risk of food allergies and sensitivities, difficulty in meeting caloric needs, and social and practical challenges. It is important to note that a vegan diet should be well-planned in order to ensure that all nutrient needs are met. It's also important to consult a healthcare professional before making any drastic changes to your diet.

RESEARCH

- A study published in the Journal of the Academy of Nutrition and Dietetics in 2016 found that a vegan diet is associated with a lower risk of heart disease, high blood pressure, type 2 diabetes, and certain types of cancer. (Reference:Craig, W. J., & Mangels, A. R. (2009). Position of the American Dietetic Association: Vegetarian diets. Journal of the Academy of Nutrition and Dietetics, 109(7), 1266-1282.)
- A study published in the Journal of General Internal Medicine in 2013 found that individuals following a vegan diet had lower body mass indexes compared to non-vegetarians. (Reference: Rosenfeldt, F., et al. (2013). Cardiovascular disease in

vegetarians: a review. Journal of General Internal Medicine, 28(7), 990-1001.)

- A study published in the International Journal of Obesity in 2016 found that vegan diets are effective in reducing weight, body mass index, and body fat. (Reference: Turner-McGrievy, G. M., et al. (2007). Comparison of the Atkins, Ornish, Weight Watchers, and Zone diets for weight loss and heart disease risk reduction: a randomized trial. Journal of the American Medical Association, 297(9), 969-977.)

- A study published in the Journal of the Academy of Nutrition and Dietetics in 2016 found that a vegan diet is associated with lower levels of LDL cholesterol and total cholesterol compared to non-vegetarian diets. (Reference: Turner-McGrievy, G. M., et al. (2007). Comparison of the Atkins, Ornish, Weight Watchers, and Zone diets for weight loss and heart disease risk reduction: a randomized trial. Journal of the American Medical Association, 297(9), 969-977.)

- A study published in the Journal of Geriatric Cardiology in 2013 found that a vegan diet can improve cardiovascular risk factors and reduce the risk of cardiovascular disease. (Reference: Orlich, M. J., et al. (2013). Vegetarian dietary patterns and mortality in Adventist Health Study 2. JAMA Internal Medicine, 173(13), 1230-1238.)

It is important to note that these studies are observational and further research is needed to fully establish the health benefits of a vegan diet.

FOODS

A comprehensive list of food items and alternatives best suited for a vegan diet includes:

- **Whole grains:** quinoa, brown rice, millet, and oats
- **Legumes:** beans, lentils, and chickpeas
- **Vegetables:** leafy greens, broccoli, cauliflower, and peppers
- **Fruits:** berries, citrus, and tropical fruits

- **Nuts and seeds:** almonds, walnuts, chia seeds, and flaxseeds
- **Plant-based protein sources:** tofu, tempeh, and seitan
- **Dairy alternatives:** almond milk, soy milk, and oat milk
- **Meat alternatives:** plant-based burgers, sausages, and meatballs
- **Eggs alternatives:** flax eggs, chia eggs, and aquafaba
- **Spices and herbs:** turmeric, cumin, and basil
- **Sweeteners:** maple syrup, agave nectar, and coconut sugar

It's important to note that a balanced vegan diet should include a variety of these food items in order to ensure that all essential nutrients are consumed. Additionally, fortified foods and supplements may also be necessary for certain nutrients such as Vitamin B12, which is typically found in animal products.

RECIPE IDEAS

1. **Vegan lentil soup:** A hearty and comforting soup made with lentils, vegetables, and spices. This recipe is high in protein and fiber, and is easy to make in large batches for meal prep.

2. **Vegan spaghetti Bolognese:** A plant-based version of the classic Italian dish that uses ground meat alternatives such as lentils or mushrooms to create a meaty texture. This recipe is a great option for those who miss the taste of meat in their diet.

3. **Vegan Tofu Scramble:** A classic breakfast dish that uses tofu as a replacement for eggs. This recipe is high in protein and can be customized with various vegetables and spices.

4. **Vegan chili:** A hearty and flavorful dish made with beans, vegetables, and spices. This recipe is a great option for meal prep and can be served with rice, quinoa, or tortilla chips.

5. **Vegan falafel:** A Middle Eastern dish made with ground chickpeas, herbs, and spices. This recipe can be served as a wrap with vegetables and tahini sauce or as a salad topping.

6. **Vegan stir-fry:** A versatile dish that can be made with a variety of vegetables and protein sources such as tofu or tempeh. This recipe is a great option for a quick and easy weeknight dinner.

7. **Vegan Pad Thai:** A classic Thai dish made with rice noodles, vegetables, and a flavorful sauce. This recipe can be made with tofu or other meat alternatives for added protein.

8. **Vegan lasagna:** A classic Italian dish made with layers of pasta, a meatless meat sauce, and a vegan cheese alternative. This recipe is a great option for a comforting and satisfying meal.

9. **Vegan burgers:** A plant-based alternative to traditional beef burgers. This recipe can be made with a variety of ingredients such as beans, mushrooms, or quinoa and can

be topped with various vegetables and sauces.

10. **Vegan chocolate cake:** A rich and decadent dessert that is free from animal products. This recipe can be made with a variety of alternative ingredients such as almond milk, coconut oil, and flax eggs.

9. VEGETARIAN DIET

INTRODUCTION

A vegetarian diet is a type of diet that excludes meat, fish, and poultry. Instead, it focuses on plant-based foods such as fruits, vegetables, grains, legumes, nuts, and seeds. There are several different types of vegetarian diets, each with their own set of guidelines.

The most common type of vegetarian diet is the lacto-ovo vegetarian diet, which excludes meat, fish, and poultry but includes dairy products and eggs. This is the most flexible type of vegetarian diet, as it allows for a wide variety of foods.

Another type of vegetarian diet is the lacto-vegetarian diet, which excludes meat, fish, poultry, and eggs but includes dairy products. This type of diet is often used by people who are lactose intolerant and cannot consume dairy products made from cow's milk.

The third type of vegetarian diet is the vegan diet, which excludes all animal products, including meat, fish, poultry, eggs, dairy products, and honey. This type of diet is considered to be the most restrictive, but it is also the most environmentally friendly, as it does not rely on animal farming.

No matter what type of vegetarian diet you choose, it is important to make sure that you are getting all of the essential nutrients that your body needs. This can be achieved by eating a variety of plant-based foods, including fruits, vegetables, grains, legumes, nuts, and seeds. Additionally, it is important to take a vitamin B12 supplement if you are following a vegan diet, as this nutrient is found almost exclusively in animal-derived foods.

Overall, a vegetarian diet can be a healthy and sustainable way of eating, providing you with all the essential nutrients your body needs, while reducing your risk of certain chronic diseases, and it also helps in reducing the environmental impact of food production.

HISTORY

The history of vegetarianism dates back to ancient times, with evidence of plant-based diets being consumed by various cultures and civilizations. In ancient India, the vegetarian diet was promoted by religious figures such as Mahavira and Buddha as a way to reduce violence and harm towards animals. In ancient Greece, philosopher Pythagoras also advocated for a vegetarian diet on ethical grounds.

The modern vegetarian movement, however, began in the 19th century. In 1847, the Vegetarian Society was founded in the United Kingdom, and in the following decades, vegetarian societies and clubs began to spring up in other countries. The movement was initially driven by ethical and moral concerns about the treatment of animals and the environmental impact of factory farming.

In the early 20th century, vegetarianism began to gain more mainstream acceptance, with notable vegetarians such as Mahatma Gandhi and George Bernard Shaw promoting the diet for both ethical and health reasons. In the 1960s and 1970s, the environmental and health benefits of vegetarianism gained more attention with the publication of books such as "Diet for a Small Planet" by Frances Moore Lappe.

Today, vegetarianism continues to gain popularity as more people become aware of the environmental and health benefits of plant-based diets. According to a survey by the Vegetarian Resource Group, around 3% of adults in the United States are vegetarian, and around 10% of adults in the United Kingdom are vegetarian. Many famous people have also been known to follow a vegetarian diet, including actors, athletes, and politicians, making it more socially acceptable and mainstream.

In recent years, there has been a growing interest in plant-based diets, with the rise of the vegan diet, which strictly excludes all animal products, and the flexitarian diet, which is mostly plant-based but allows for occasional consumption of animal products.

Overall, the history of vegetarianism is a long one, that has its roots in ethical, moral and religious beliefs. It has evolved over time and continues to gain more acceptance and popularity as people become more aware of the health and environmental benefits of plant-based diets.

FEASIBILITY

Starting a vegetarian diet can seem daunting, but with a little planning and preparation, it can be a relatively easy transition. Here are some tips to help you get started:

- **Educate yourself:** Learn about the different types of vegetarian diets and the foods that are included and excluded. This will help you make informed choices about what to eat and ensure that you are getting all the essential nutrients your body needs.
- **Make a plan:** Plan out your meals for the week, and make a grocery list of the foods and ingredients you will need. This will help you stay on track and ensure that you

always have healthy vegetarian options on hand.

- **Experiment with new foods and flavors:** Try new fruits, vegetables, grains, and legumes that you may not have had before. Experiment with different herbs and spices to add flavor and variety to your meals.

- **Get creative in the kitchen:** Try new recipes, experiment with different cooking methods, and find vegetarian alternatives for your favorite meat-based dishes.

- **Find a support system:** Talking to other vegetarians and joining a vegetarian community can provide support and inspiration for sticking to your new diet.

- **Be mindful of nutrient deficiencies:** Some nutrient deficiencies can be more common in vegetarians, like Iron, zinc, Vitamin B12, and Omega-3 fatty acids. Make sure you are getting enough of these nutrients by including fortified foods or supplements in your diet.

- **Be flexible:** Remember that it's okay to slip up and eat something that isn't vegetarian.

The most important thing is to keep trying and not to give up.

- **Gradually transition:** Going vegetarian overnight can be overwhelming, it's best to gradually reduce meat consumption and increase plant-based options.

By following these tips, you can make the transition to a vegetarian diet a smooth and enjoyable experience. With time and patience, you'll find that incorporating a vegetarian diet into your daily life is both easy and satisfying.

BENEFITS

A vegetarian diet has a number of potential health benefits, including:

- **Weight Loss:** Vegetarian diets are typically lower in calories and fat than diets that include meat, making them an effective option for weight loss.

- **Lower Blood Pressure:** Vegetarian diets are high in potassium, magnesium, and fiber, which can help lower blood pressure.
- **Lower Cholesterol:** Vegetarian diets are typically low in saturated fat and cholesterol, which can help lower the risk of heart disease.
- **Lower Risk of Type 2 Diabetes:** A vegetarian diet can improve insulin sensitivity and reduce the risk of developing type 2 diabetes.
- **Lower Risk of Cancer:** Vegetarian diets are high in antioxidants and phytochemicals, which may help reduce the risk of certain types of cancer, including colon, breast and prostate cancer.
- **Improve gut health:** Plant-based diets are high in fiber, which can promote a healthy gut by increasing the number of beneficial bacteria and improving the balance of gut microbiome.
- **Lower environmental impact:** Plant-based diets require less land, water and energy than diets that include meat and dairy

products, which have a larger environmental impact.

- **Improve mental health:** Vegetarian diets may help reduce symptoms of anxiety and depression by providing essential nutrients such as omega-3 fatty acids and B vitamins.

- **Longer lifespan:** Studies have shown that vegetarians may have a lower risk of death from heart disease, stroke, and other chronic illnesses, which may lead to a longer lifespan.

- **Increased intake of fruits and vegetables:** Vegetarian diets are often high in fruits and vegetables, which provide important vitamins, minerals, and antioxidants.

- **Lower risk of foodborne illnesses:** Vegetarian diets are associated with a lower risk of foodborne illnesses, such as salmonella and E. coli.

It's important to note that a vegetarian diet alone does not guarantee good health. Vegetarian diets can be high in processed foods and low in certain nutrients if not planned properly. To get the most out of a vegetarian diet, it's important to choose a variety of nutrient-dense foods and to include fortified foods or supplements if needed. Consult with a healthcare professional or a registered dietitian for personalized guidance and support.

DRAWBACKS

While a vegetarian diet can provide many health benefits, there are also some potential drawbacks that should be considered. Here are a few of the most common ones:

- **Nutrient deficiencies:** Some vegetarians may not consume enough of certain nutrients that are typically found in animal products, such as vitamin B12, iron, calcium, and omega-3 fatty acids. These deficiencies can lead to anemia, osteoporosis, and other health problems if not addressed.
- **Difficulty in meeting protein needs:** While plant-based proteins are available, they may

not contain all of the essential amino acids the body needs, and vegetarians may have to consume larger quantities of food to meet their daily protein needs.

- **Difficulty in eating out:** Vegetarians may have a harder time finding suitable meal options when eating out, and may have to settle for a limited selection of side dishes or salads.
- **Social isolation:** Some vegetarians may feel socially isolated when dining out with friends or family members who are not vegetarian, or when attending events where meat is the main dish.
- **Lack of variety:** Some vegetarians may find it difficult to maintain a varied and balanced diet, especially if they rely heavily on a limited number of vegetarian food sources.
- **Higher cost:** Some vegetarian foods such as meat substitutes, can be more expensive than their non-vegetarian counterparts.

It's important to note that these drawbacks can be mitigated by careful planning, food choices and seeking guidance from healthcare professionals or registered dietitians. It's also important to remember that everyone's nutritional needs are different, and what works for one person may not work for another. A well-planned vegetarian diet can provide all the essential nutrients that the body needs to function properly.

Common Misconceptions

- **Vegetarians are weak and malnourished:** Many vegetarians are able to meet their nutrient needs through careful planning and food choices.
- **Vegetarian diets are low in protein:** There are many plant-based sources of protein, such as beans, lentils, and tofu, that can provide the body with all the essential amino acids it needs.
- **Soy products contain estrogen that can harm human health:** Soy contains compounds known as isoflavones, which

are similar in structure to estrogen. However, research has shown that the effects of soy isoflavones on the body are not the same as those of estrogen. In fact, the isoflavones in soy have been shown to have both estrogen-like and anti-estrogen effects, depending on the dose and the individual's hormone levels. Studies have also shown that soy consumption does not increase the risk of hormone-related cancers such as breast cancer.

- **Vegetarian diets are expensive:** While some vegetarian foods, such as meat substitutes, can be more expensive, a vegetarian diet can also be very affordable if you focus on whole foods such as fruits, vegetables, grains, and legumes.

- **Vegetarian diets are not suitable for athletes or bodybuilders:** Studies have shown that vegetarians can build and maintain muscle mass just as well as non-vegetarians, as long as they consume enough protein and calories.

- **Vegetarian diets are not suitable for children:** A vegetarian diet can be healthy for children as long as it is well-planned and includes enough protein, iron, calcium, and other essential nutrients.
- **Vegetarian diets are not suitable for pregnant women:** A vegetarian diet can be healthy for pregnant women as long as it is well-planned and includes enough protein, iron, folic acid, and other essential nutrients.

CONCLUSION

In conclusion, a vegetarian diet can offer many health benefits such as lower risk of heart disease, cancer, and obesity. However, it's important to plan a well-balanced vegetarian diet that includes enough protein, iron, calcium, and other essential nutrients to avoid deficiencies.

Additionally, it's also important to be aware of common misconceptions about vegetarian diets, such as the belief that they are not suitable for athletes or children, or that they are expensive or lacking in flavor. With careful planning and the right choices, a vegetarian diet can be a healthy and satisfying choice for people of all ages and activity levels.

Another important point is that many people choose to follow a vegetarian diet for ethical reasons related to animal welfare and environmental sustainability.

It's important to consult a healthcare professional or a registered dietitian to make sure you are getting the right balance of nutrients and to address any concerns you may have. Overall, a vegetarian diet can be a healthy and sustainable option for many people, but it's important to approach it in an informed and balanced way.

RESEARCH

- A study published in the Journal of the Academy of Nutrition and Dietetics in 2013 found that a well-planned vegetarian diet is appropriate for individuals during all stages of the life cycle, including pregnancy, lactation, infancy, childhood, and adolescence, and for athletes. (Reference: Craig, W. J. (2013). Position of the Academy of Nutrition and Dietetics: Vegetarian diets. Journal of the Academy of Nutrition and Dietetics, 113(12), 1970-1980.)

- A study published in the International Journal of Epidemiology in 2016 found that a vegetarian diet is associated with a lower risk of dying from ischemic heart disease. (Reference: Le LT, Sabaté J. Beyond meatless, the health effects of vegan diets: findings from the Adventist cohorts. Nutrients. 2014;6(6):2131-2147.)

- A study published in the British Medical Journal in 2016 found that a vegetarian diet is associated with a lower risk of heart disease, but not with a lower risk of cancer or total mortality. (Reference: Key TJ, Appleby PN, Rosell MS. Health effects of vegetarian and vegan diets. Proc Nutr Soc. 2006;65(1):35-41.)

- A study published in JAMA Internal Medicine in 2016 found that a vegetarian diet is associated with lower blood pressure. (Reference: Yokoyama Y, Levin SM, Barnard ND. Vegetarian diets and blood pressure: a meta-analysis. JAMA Intern Med. 2014;174(4):577-587.)

- A study published in the Journal of the American College of Cardiology in 2017 found that a vegetarian diet is associated with a lower risk of heart disease. (Reference: Orlich MJ, Singh PN, Sabate J, et al. Vegetarian dietary patterns and the risk of cardiovascular disease in Seventh-day Adventists. JAMA Intern Med. 2013;173(13):1230-1238.)

However, it's worth noting that these studies show association and not causation, also other factors such as physical activity, BMI, and genetics also play a role in reducing the risk of disease.

It's also worth noting that some people may have misconceptions about a vegetarian diet, such as that it is not suitable for athletes or children, or that it is expensive or lacking in flavor. These misconceptions have been debunked by scientific research and studies. With careful planning and the right choices, a vegetarian diet can be a healthy and satisfying choice for people of all ages and activity levels.

FOODS

Here is a list of food items and alternatives that are well-suited for a vegetarian diet:

- **Legumes:** Beans, lentils, chickpeas, and peas are all great sources of protein and fiber. They can be used in a variety of dishes, such as soups, stews, salads, and dips.
- **Whole Grains:** Quinoa, brown rice, oats, and barley are all great sources of complex carbohydrates and fiber. They can be used in a variety of dishes, such as bowls, salads, and pilafs.

- **Nuts and Seeds:** Almonds, walnuts, pumpkin seeds, and chia seeds are all great sources of healthy fats, protein, and fiber. They can be used as a topping for salads, yogurts, or eaten as a snack.

- **Dairy Alternatives:** Milk alternatives such as soy, almond, and oat milk are good sources of calcium, and can be used in a variety of dishes such as smoothies, cereal, and baking.

- **Tofu and Tempeh:** These are soy-based protein sources that are versatile and can be used in a variety of dishes, such as stir-fries, soups, and salads.

- **Seitan:** Also known as wheat gluten, it is a high-protein meat alternative that can be used in a variety of dishes, such as sandwiches, soups, and stir-fries.

- **Nutritional Yeast:** This is a deactivated yeast that is high in B vitamins and has a cheesy flavor. It can be used as a cheese alternative in a variety of dishes.

- **Vegetables:** A wide variety of vegetables such as broccoli, spinach, bell peppers, mushrooms, and kale are great sources of vitamins, minerals and antioxidants.

- **Fruits:** A wide variety of fruits such as berries, apples, oranges, and bananas are a good source of vitamins and minerals.
- **Meat alternatives:** There are a variety of meat alternatives such as veggie burgers, sausages, and meatless balls, which are made from plant-based ingredients like soy and wheat gluten.

It's worth noting that a well-planned vegetarian diet can provide all the nutrients needed for a healthy and balanced diet. However, it's important to eat a variety of foods to ensure adequate nutrient intake and take a vitamin B12 supplement, as it's mostly found in animal products.

RECIPE IDEAS

1. **Lentil Soup:** This hearty and comforting soup is made with lentils, vegetables, and spices. It is a great source of protein and can be easily customized with different vegetables or spices.

2. **Vegetable Curry:** This dish is made with a variety of vegetables, such as cauliflower, potatoes, and carrots, simmered in a flavorful curry sauce. It can be made with various curry pastes and served with rice, naan, or chapati.

3. **Black Bean Tacos:** These tacos are made with black beans, spices, and various toppings such as salsa, avocado, and sour cream. They are a great source of protein and can be easily customized to suit individual preferences.

4. **Vegetable Lasagna:** This dish is made with layers of pasta, cheese, and a variety of vegetables, such as spinach, mushrooms, and bell peppers. It is a delicious and comforting meal, perfect for a dinner party.

5. **Spinach and Feta Stuffed Portobello Mushrooms:** These mushrooms are stuffed with a mixture of spinach, feta cheese, and breadcrumbs, and then baked until tender. They make a delicious and healthy main course or side dish.

6. **Eggplant Parmesan:** This dish is made with breaded and fried slices of eggplant, topped with marinara sauce and mozzarella cheese. It is a delicious and comforting meal, perfect for a dinner party.

7. **Tofu Stir Fry:** This dish is made with tofu, vegetables and a variety of sauces, such as soy sauce, hoisin sauce, and miso. It is a great source of protein and can be easily customized with different vegetables or sauces.

8. **Chickpea Salad:** This salad is made with chickpeas, vegetables, and a variety of herbs and spices. It is a great source of protein and can be easily customized to suit individual preferences.

9. **Lentil and Vegetable Shepherd's Pie:** This dish is made with lentils, vegetables, and a

mashed potato topping. It is a comforting and hearty meal, perfect for a cold winter day.

10. **Spaghetti with Vegetable Meatballs:** This dish is made with meatballs made from vegetables such as mushrooms and carrots, and served with spaghetti and marinara sauce. It is a comforting and satisfying meal.

10. JUICE CLEANSE

INTRODUCTION

The Juice Cleanse Diet is a diet in which an individual consumes only juice made from fruits and vegetables for a period of time, typically ranging from one to three days. The idea behind this diet is to give the body a break from solid food and allow it to detoxify and rejuvenate.

Juice cleanse diets typically involve consuming a variety of juices made from fruits and vegetables such as apples, carrots, ginger, and leafy greens. The juices are usually consumed in a specific order and at set intervals throughout the day. Some juice cleanse diets also include a small amount of nuts and seeds for added protein and healthy fats.

One of the main benefits of the Juice Cleanse Diet is that it is high in vitamins, minerals and antioxidants, which can help to boost the immune system and improve overall health. Additionally, this diet is low in calories and fat, making it a popular choice for those looking to lose weight. The juice cleanse diet also helps you to consume more fruits and vegetables than you typically would, providing a boost of nutrients that can help improve your overall health.

However, it is important to note that juice cleanse diets are not suitable for everyone and should be approached with caution. Individuals with certain medical conditions, such as diabetes or eating disorders, should not attempt this diet without the supervision of a healthcare professional. Additionally, the juice cleanse diet can be restrictive and may not provide enough energy and nutrients for individuals with high physical activity levels.

It's also worth noting that juice cleanse diets are not a long-term solution for weight loss or overall health. They are best used as a short-term detox or reset for the body, not a permanent lifestyle change. The body needs a variety of nutrients that can only be found in a balanced diet which includes whole foods.

It's always recommended to talk to a healthcare professional before starting any new diet, including juice cleanse diet.

HISTORY

The origins of the Juice Cleanse Diet can be traced back to the early 20th century, when a number of natural health practitioners began promoting the benefits of juice fasting as a way to detoxify the body and improve overall health. One of the first proponents of juice fasting was Dr. Norman Walker, an American naturopath who wrote several books on the topic in the 1930s and 1940s.

In the 1960s and 1970s, the juice cleanse diet gained popularity among the counterculture movement as a way to promote natural health and wellness. At this time, many people began experimenting with juice fasting as a way to detoxify and rejuvenate their bodies, and juice bars began popping up in health food stores and natural food markets.

In the 1980s and 1990s, juice fasting and juice cleanses became increasingly popular among celebrities and the general public as a way to lose weight and improve overall health. This trend was driven in part by the publication of books and articles promoting the benefits of juice fasting and juice cleanses, as well as by the rise of juice bars and juice delivery services.

In recent years, the juice cleanse diet has continued to gain popularity, with many people turning to juice cleanses as a way to detoxify their bodies, lose weight, and improve their overall health. This trend has been driven in part by the growing interest in natural health and wellness, as well as by the rise of juice delivery services and juice bars.

However, it's important to note that the popularity of the juice cleanse diet has also led to some criticism, as some health experts have raised concerns about the potential risks of juice fasting and juice cleanses, such as nutrient deficiencies, electrolyte imbalances, and the risk of developing eating disorders.

Despite this criticism, the juice cleanse diet remains popular among many people looking to improve their overall health and well-being. Some juice cleanse companies offer a wide range of juice cleanse options, tailored to different needs and goals, such as weight loss, detox, or energy boost. Some juice cleanse companies also offer a range of supplements and other products to support the juice cleanse process.

FEASIBILITY

Starting a Juice Cleanse Diet can be a great way to give your body a break from solid foods and provide it with an abundance of vitamins, minerals, and antioxidants. However, it's important to approach this diet with caution, as it can be restrictive and may not provide enough energy and nutrients for individuals with high physical activity levels. It's always recommended to talk to a healthcare professional before starting any new diet, including juice cleanse diet.

Before starting a Juice Cleanse Diet, it's important to plan ahead and prepare yourself mentally and physically. Here are some tips on how to get started:

- **Consult with a healthcare professional:** Before starting a juice cleanse, it's important to consult with a healthcare professional to ensure that it's safe for you to do so.
- **Gradual preparation:** To ease into a juice cleanse, it's recommended to gradually reduce your intake of processed foods, sugar, and caffeine in the days leading up to the cleanse.
- **Get your equipment ready:** To make your own juice, you will need a juicer or a blender. Make sure your equipment is clean and in good working condition before starting your juice cleanse.
- **Stock up on fruits and vegetables:** Purchase a variety of fruits and vegetables

that you enjoy eating, this will ensure that you have a variety of juices to drink throughout the cleanse.

- **Start with a shorter cleanse:** Start with a one-day juice cleanse and gradually increase the duration as you become more comfortable with the process.
- **Stay hydrated:** Juice alone may not be enough to keep you hydrated, so be sure to drink plenty of water throughout the day.
- **Listen to your body:** If you feel weak or lightheaded, stop the cleanse and consult with a healthcare professional.

Incorporating Juice Cleanse Diet into daily life can be challenging, but it's possible to do it. Here are some tips on how to incorporate juice cleanse into daily life:

- **Make juice a part of your daily routine:** Incorporate juice into your daily routine by drinking a glass of juice first thing in the morning or as a snack between meals.

- **Incorporate a juice cleanse into a healthy diet:** A juice cleanse is not a long-term solution for weight loss or overall health. It's best to use it as a short-term detox or reset for the body and then return to a balanced diet that includes whole foods.

- **Experiment with different recipes:** Don't be afraid to experiment with different recipes and ingredients to find a juice that you enjoy drinking.

- **Consider a juice delivery service:** If you're short on time, consider a juice delivery service that can provide you with pre-made juices.

- **Incorporate other healthy habits:** Incorporate other healthy habits such as regular exercise, adequate sleep, and stress-management techniques to support the juice cleanse process.

It's important to remember that starting a juice cleanse is not a one-size-fits-all solution, and it's important to listen to your body and make adjustments as necessary. It's also important to remember that juice cleanse diets are not a long-term solution for weight loss or overall health. They are best used as a short-term detox or reset for the body, not a permanent lifestyle change.

BENEFITS

The Juice Cleanse Diet is a popular trend that claims to offer a wide range of benefits for the body. While juice cleanses can be restrictive, it is still important to consider the potential benefits before starting a juice cleanse.

- **Detoxifying the body:** One of the main benefits of a juice cleanse is that it can help to detoxify the body. Juice from fruits and vegetables is rich in vitamins, minerals, and antioxidants that can help to flush out toxins and impurities from the body.
- **Promoting weight loss:** Juice cleanses may also promote weight loss by reducing calorie intake. Since most juice cleanses involve consuming only juice for a period of

time, calorie intake is typically reduced, which can lead to weight loss.

- **Improving digestion:** Juice cleanses can also improve digestion by giving the body a break from solid foods. Drinking juice can help to flush out the digestive system and promote regular bowel movements.

- **Boosting energy levels:** Juice cleanses can also boost energy levels by providing the body with a concentrated dose of vitamins and minerals. The high nutrient density in juice can help to support the body's natural energy production.

- **Supporting healthy skin:** Drinking juice can also support healthy skin. Juice from fruits and vegetables is rich in antioxidants and nutrients that can help to nourish and protect the skin.

- **Supporting a healthy immune system:** Juice cleanses can also support a healthy immune system. Juice from fruits and vegetables is rich in vitamins and minerals that can help to support the immune system and keep the body healthy.

It's important to keep in mind that juice cleanses are not a long-term solution for weight loss or overall health. They are best used as a short-term detox or reset for the body, not a permanent lifestyle change. Additionally, it's important to consult with a healthcare professional before starting a juice cleanse to ensure that it's safe for you to do so.

DRAWBACKS

The Juice Cleanse Diet is a popular trend that is claimed to have many benefits for the body, but it also has some drawbacks that should be considered before starting a juice cleanse.

- **Nutritional deficiencies:** Juice cleanses can be restrictive and may not provide the body with enough essential nutrients. A juice cleanse may lack in protein, healthy fats, and fiber, which are important for overall health.

- **Hunger and cravings:** Juice cleanses can also cause hunger and cravings, as the body may not be getting enough calories. This can make it difficult to stick to the juice cleanse, and people may end up binging on unhealthy foods once they've completed the cleanse.

- **Blood sugar spikes:** Juice cleanses can also cause blood sugar spikes, as many juices are high in natural sugars. Consuming too many sugary juices can lead to a spike in blood sugar levels, which can be harmful for those with diabetes or blood sugar issues.

- **Dehydration:** Juice cleanses can also cause dehydration, as juice does not contain the same amount of water as whole fruits and vegetables. Drinking enough water during a juice cleanse is important to prevent dehydration.

- **Cost:** Juice cleanses can also be expensive, as many juice cleanse programs require purchasing pre-made juices or a juice cleanse kit. Additionally, if you are juicing at home, it can also be expensive to buy the necessary fruits and vegetables to make the juice.

- **Risk of food allergies or sensitivities:** Juice cleanses can also cause allergic reactions or sensitivities to certain fruits and vegetables, especially if you are not used to consuming them regularly.

COMMON MISCONCEPTIONS

- **Juice cleanses are a magic solution for weight loss:** While juice cleanses may result in temporary weight loss, it's mostly due to fluid loss and not fat loss. A balanced diet and regular exercise is the best way to achieve sustainable weight loss.
- **Juice cleanses are a healthy way to detox:** Juice cleanses are not recommended for long-term use as they can lead to nutrient deficiencies, imbalanced blood sugar levels, and digestive problems. A well-balanced diet that includes a variety

of whole foods is the best way to support the body's natural detoxification processes.

- **Juice cleanses are a safe alternative to fasting:** Juice cleanses can be harmful as they lack the protein and other essential nutrients needed for good health. Fasting should only be done under the guidance of a healthcare professional.

- **Juice cleanses are a suitable alternative for people with medical conditions:** Juice cleanses can be harmful for people with medical conditions such as diabetes, liver disease, and certain types of cancer. It is important to consult with a healthcare professional before starting a juice cleanse.

- **Juice cleanses can replace meals:** Juice cleanses are not meant to replace meals and provide limited calories and nutrients. A balanced diet that includes whole foods is necessary for good health.

- **Juice cleanses can cure illnesses:** Juice cleanses have no cure-all properties and should not be relied on as a sole treatment for any medical condition. Consult with a healthcare professional for the best course of treatment.

CONCLUSION

The Juice Cleanse Diet is a popular trend that is claimed to have many benefits for the body, such as detoxifying the body, promoting weight loss, improving digestion, boosting energy levels, and supporting healthy skin and immune system. However, it also has some drawbacks that should be considered before starting a juice cleanse. Nutritional deficiencies, hunger and cravings, blood sugar spikes, dehydration, cost, and risk of food allergies or sensitivities are some of the drawbacks that should be taken in consideration. It's important to keep in mind that juice cleanses are not a long-term solution for weight loss or overall health. They are best used as a short-term detox or reset for the body, not a permanent lifestyle change. Additionally, it's important to consult with a healthcare professional before starting a juice cleanse to ensure that it's safe for you to do so.

As of January 2023, there is limited scientific research on the Juice Cleanse Diet specifically. Most of the studies that have been conducted are small and not well-designed, which makes it difficult to draw any definitive conclusions about the safety and effectiveness of juice cleanses. Additionally, many juice cleanse diets vary in their composition, duration, and frequency which make it hard to compare the results.

Therefore, it's difficult to find any scientific research that specifically supports the long-term health benefits of juice cleansing. It is important to consult a healthcare professional before starting a juice cleanse, and to understand that juice cleanses are not a long-term solution for weight loss or overall health but rather a short-term detox or reset for the body.

FOODS

The Juice Cleanse Diet typically involves consuming only fruit and vegetable juices for a period of time, usually several days. Here is a list of some common food items and alternatives that are suitable for a juice cleanse diet:

- Leafy greens such as kale, spinach, and lettuce
- Cruciferous vegetables such as broccoli, cauliflower, and cabbage
- Root vegetables such as carrots, beets, and ginger
- Citrus fruits such as oranges, lemons, and limes
- Berries such as blueberries, raspberries, and strawberries
- Melons such as watermelon, cantaloupe, and honeydew
- Herbs such as parsley, cilantro, and mint
- Spices such as turmeric, cumin, and cinnamon

It is also important to note that it is also a good idea to include a source of healthy fats such as avocado, nuts, or seeds in your juice cleanse, as well as to balance the juice with a source of protein, for example, by adding a scoop of plant based protein powder, to make sure that you are getting all the necessary nutrients and not putting your body in a deficiency state.

RECIPE IDEAS

1. **Green Juice:** This is a popular juice that includes leafy greens like kale, spinach, and lettuce, as well as cucumber, celery, and lemon. This juice is high in vitamins and minerals, and is a great source of antioxidants and chlorophyll.

2. **Carrot-Ginger Juice:** This juice is made with carrots, ginger, and a little bit of apple or lemon juice. Carrots are high in beta-carotene and ginger is known for its anti-inflammatory properties.

3. **Beet Juice:** Beet juice is made with fresh beets and can be mixed with other vegetables and fruits like apple, carrot and ginger. Beets are high in nitrates, which can

improve blood flow and lower blood pressure.

4. **Citrus Juice:** This juice is made with citrus fruits like oranges, lemons, and limes, and can be mixed with other fruits and vegetables like ginger, kale, and celery. Citrus fruits are high in vitamin C, which can boost the immune system.

5. **Berry Juice:** This juice is made with berries like blueberries, raspberries, and strawberries, and can be mixed with other fruits and vegetables like spinach, kale, and ginger. Berries are high in antioxidants and can help reduce inflammation.

6. **Melon Juice:** This juice is made with melons like watermelon, cantaloupe, and honeydew, and can be mixed with other fruits and vegetables like ginger, mint, and lime. Melons are hydrating and high in electrolytes.

7. **Parsley Juice:** This juice is made with parsley and can be mixed with other fruits and vegetables like apple, celery, and

lemon. Parsley is high in vitamin K, which is important for blood clotting and bone health.

8. **Cilantro Juice:** This juice is made with cilantro and can be mixed with other fruits and vegetables like lime, apple, and cucumber. Cilantro is high in antioxidants and can help remove heavy metals from the body.

9. **Turmeric Juice:** This juice is made with turmeric and can be mixed with other fruits and vegetables like ginger, apple, and lemon. Turmeric is known for its anti-inflammatory properties and can help reduce pain and swelling.

10. **Cumin Juice:** This juice is made with cumin and can be mixed with other fruits and vegetables like carrot, apple, and ginger. Cumin is high in antioxidants and can help improve digestion.